AF768768

Better Living and Breathing

A MANUAL FOR PATIENTS

Better Living and Breathing

A MANUAL FOR PATIENTS

Kenneth M. Moser, M.D.
Carol Archibald, R.N.
Patsy Hansen, R.N.
Birgitta Ellis, P.T.
Donna Whelan, R.R.T.

Pulmonary Division, University of California, San Diego

SECOND EDITION

with 129 illustrations by **Steve Pileggi**

This book has been approved by the Publications Subcommittee of the American Thoracic Society's Medical Education Committee.

The C. V. Mosby Company

ST. LOUIS • TORONTO • LONDON 1980

SECOND EDITION

Copyright © 1980 by The C. V. Mosby Company

All rights reserved. No part of this book may be reproduced in any manner without written permission of the publisher.

Previous edition copyrighted 1975

Printed in the United States of America

The C. V. Mosby Company
11830 Westline Industrial Drive, St. Louis, Missouri 63141

Library of Congress Cataloging in Publication Data

Main entry under title:

Better living and breathing.

Bibliography: p.
Includes index.
1. Lungs—Diseases, Obstructive. 2. Health attitudes. I. Moser, Kenneth M. [DNLM: 1. Lung diseases, Obstructive—Popular works. WF600 B565]
RC776.03B37 1980 616.2′4 80-17943
ISBN 0-8016-3565-9

VT/M/M 9 8 7 6 5 4 3 2 01/C/040

Foreword

Breathing is a function that is taken for granted by everyone except patients like yourself, who suffer from diseases of the heart or lungs. Unlike pneumonia, where antibiotics are often curative, no "miracle drug" has been discovered to completely alleviate the discomfort caused by chronic lung diseases.

By nature, these diseases—asthma, bronchitis, and emphysema—are far more complex than pneumonia and not so easily defined or cured. Because the diseases themselves are complex, their treatment is often complicated.

Most patients are taught how to care for their lung disease while in the hospital. Many of these patients forget much of what they have learned in the hectic and less ordered pace of home life. Some of them return to the hospital again and again, representing failures not so much of the therapy prescribed, but of their ability to learn the various maneuvers and procedures taught to them in the hospital.

Indeed, the most important ingredient in the successful management of chronic lung disease *has* been discovered—YOU! Working with well-trained physicians, nurses, respiratory therapists, and physical therapists, the enlightened and informed patient is a mighty weapon. If *you* have a good understanding of the respiratory system and your treatment program, you can become a vital member of your own health care team.

This manual is written to help you become a knowledgeable participant in your own rehabilitation effort. It is intended to be used by you, your doctor, and other medical personnel who assist in your care. You are all partners in better breathing and better living. When you have finished reading this little book, I would suggest that you keep it for frequent review. Share it with members of your family so they, too, can understand the complexity of your problem and what is being done to relieve it.

If this book is successful, you will be less disabled by your illness, less restricted in your activities, and, most important, able to be at home where you belong, rather than forever in the hospital. My best wishes to you for continued recovery.

George G. Burton, M.D.

Professor of Medicine, Loma Linda University,
Loma Linda, California

Preface

Any book with multiple authors of different background must have an interesting story behind it, and this one does. The story began some 15 years ago when several of us decided to develop a program based on two concepts which, at that time, were relatively new. The first was that patients with chronic pulmonary diseases could live a better life if they were educated about the anatomy, physiology, and treatment of their diseases. Such patients could then become participants in, rather than be mere observers of, the health care provided. The second concept was that such an educational effort could be provided most effectively by a respiratory care team that included individuals with a wide range of professional skills and knowledge: pulmonary physicians, pulmonary nursing specialists, respiratory therapists, chest physical therapists, cardiopulmonary technologists, psychiatrists, social workers, nutritionists, occupational therapists, and administrators.

Both of these concepts not only were rather new, they were also untested. There was concern in some quarters that the educated patient might be more of a threat than a help to the health care system, that patients would not be interested in such self-education, and that such attempts might be viewed as incursions upon doctor-patient relationships. Some wondered whether the attempts to develop such a team would founder on the rocks of interprofessional jealousy—whether "team interaction" would be more conducive to dissension than education. Despite such reservations, the effort was undertaken.

The team was developed and together designed a course for patients with chronic lung diseases. The first patients came and learned and were benefitted. The process was refined and repeated, and a gratifying dividend appeared. As the years and the courses passed, many physicians and allied health professionals attended in order to learn the course elements and begin similar efforts at their offices, clinics, and hospitals.

But an increasing source of frustration to us was that our educational efforts were still reaching a relatively small audience. Our program was consistently "backlogged," so that we could reach only a modest percentage of the patients with chronic lung disease in our immediate geographic area, and extension of our program to other areas was not feasible. This book was a logical means for extending our educational efforts to this larger patient audience that we could never personally reach. So that is the story behind the first edition of this book, which appeared in 1975. In the interval, we have continued to learn from our patients and colleagues, and some new concepts and treatments have developed. It is fitting that, as we enter a new decade, we should provide a second edition incorporating the suggestions and changes accumulated over the intervening years.

One thing, however, has not changed; indeed, it has become stronger. That is our belief that patients with chronic pulmonary disease can become active members of the treatment team, accepting (and enjoying) the fact that they can and must play a central role in their own care. That is still the theme of this book. In fact, since 1975 that has become a national theme in the area of health care: the patient's active participation in the goal of maintaining and improving his or her health.

We hope that all of our colleagues in respiratory care will continue to find this book useful and that patients with chronic pulmonary disease will learn from its pages how to live better and more functional lives.

Of course, despite the multiple authorship, many others have contributed directly or indirectly to this book. We owe special debts of gratitude to Steve Pileggi, whose illustrations have contributed so much to our programs and this book; Dr. Stephen Groban, whose devotion to the mental health of our patients has helped them (and us) live better lives; Jane Villareal, a social worker whose caring and understanding are exemplary; Joyce Knott, who has taught us all much about nutrition; Richard Levy, for sharing his expertise in pharmacology; Roseanne Myers, R.N., and Deon Dunn, R.N., whose efforts have had a major influence on our program and this volume; a succession of pulmonary trainees and students at UCSD who have been our teachers as well as our students; Paula Powell and Dena Lomax, who have borne the administrative burdens of translating our ideas to a readable copy; and, finally, our patients, who have continued to return more to us than we have given to them.

Kenneth M. Moser

Note to the reader

A number of medications, exercises, and other forms of medical treatment are reviewed in this book. While the descriptions are as accurate as possible, they should not be taken as direct instruction or recommendation for any individual patient. The contents of this book are informational only. Any specific medication or exercise should be prescribed by a physician and initiated under appropriate medical guidance.

Contents

Better Living and Breathing

A MANUAL FOR PATIENTS

1 The lungs: how they are put together and how they work

In order to understand your disease, you should know how normal lungs are built and how they work. Then it is easier to recognize what has happened to your lungs, why you get certain symptoms, and what you and your doctor can do to improve these symptoms. There is some new vocabulary involved. If you learn these new words, you will be able to talk with your doctor more easily and not be confused by things he says or articles you may read about lung disease.

HOW THE BODY'S ENGINE RUNS

The human body was designed to run on oxygen as its "energy" source, just as automobile engines run on gasoline or diesel fuel and power plants run on coal, oil, or other fuels. And, just as with other fuels, when the body "burns" oxygen for energy, waste products result; the two major waste products are water and carbon dioxide.

Therefore, all of the body's functions depend on delivery of a steady supply of oxygen. Unfortunately, the body cannot store much oxygen. If delivery stops, the body "runs out of gas" (oxygen) within about 5 minutes. So the supply must be continuous, unlike the supply of food or water.

Furthermore, the waste products must be excreted promptly. Getting rid of water presents no problems. If the body retains water, it can still function and, sooner or later, excrete (get rid of) it through the kidneys as urine or through the sweat glands. But if carbon dioxide builds up in the body, it creates acids in the blood; an excess of such acids can impair the function of important organs such as the brain and heart. So a build-up of carbon dioxide can produce symptoms such as headache, drowsiness, and fatigue.

The lungs are designed to solve the twin problems of continuous oxygen delivery and carbon dioxide removal. They are the only route by which oxygen can be delivered to the body. Acids and carbon dioxide can be excreted by the kidneys, but the lungs get rid of carbon dioxide (and prevent acidity) much more quickly and efficiently than do the kidneys.

In order to carry out these two vital functions, the lungs need to have

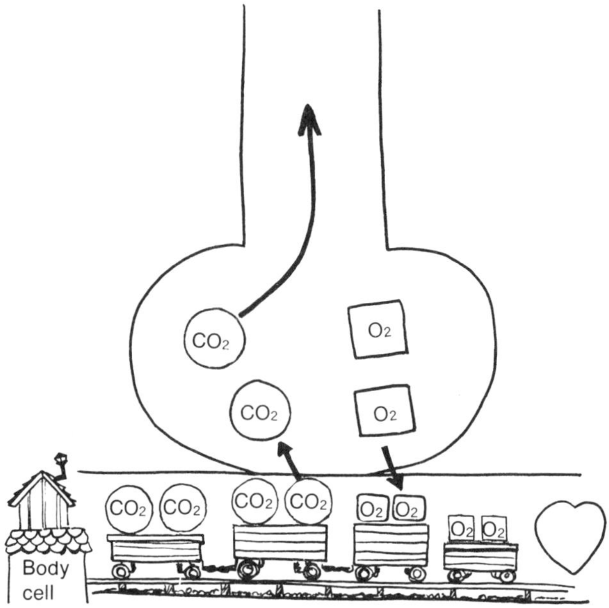

a practical way to bring fresh air (inspired air) into contact with the blood in a safe manner, so that the blood can pick up oxygen and get rid of excess carbon dioxide. Then the air must be efficiently expelled (expired) into the environment, and the blood pumped to the rest of the body.

HOW THE LUNGS ARE DESIGNED

Step one: getting air in and out

This function is carried out by a system of branching air tubes (bronchial tubes) to bring air in and out of the lungs, and a system of blood tubes (pulmonary arteries) to bring blood to the lungs. The system of air tubes is called the *bronchial tree,* an appropriate name because it looks like an upside-down tree. It begins with a single, large tube (like the tree "trunk") called the windpipe or *trachea,* which you can feel with your fingers in your neck. The trachea is the entrance to the lungs; it also contains the *larynx* (or voice box). The trachea extends from the back of the mouth to the inside of the chest (*thorax*). There the trachea divides into two major branches (one to the right lung, one to the left lung). Next, each of these *main stem bronchi* branches many times into smaller and smaller *bronchial tubes,* just as a tree branches. When the branches become very small (so small that they can be seen only with a microscope), they are given a new name: *bronchioles.* The larger bronchial tubes have *cartilage* in their walls. Cartilage is a rigid but flexible ma-

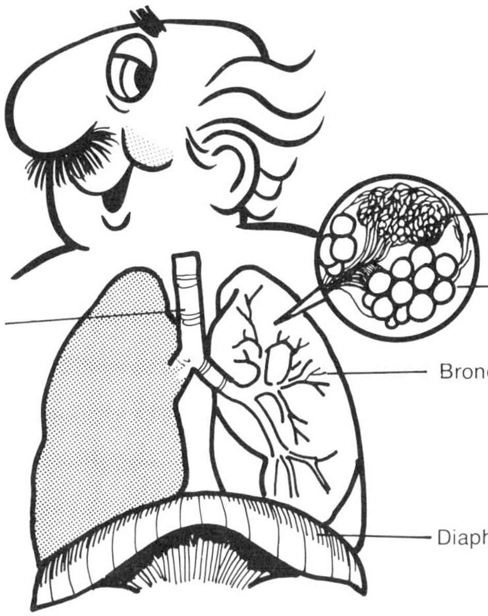

terial—flexible enough to change shape as we breathe but rigid enough to prevent the larger bronchial tubes from collapsing. The smaller bronchial tubes have no cartilage in their walls; they are surrounded by a circle of *muscle.* If this muscle contracts, the tubes can be greatly narrowed. All bronchial tubes are lined by a delicate layer of cells (the *mucous membrane*). Some of the cells in this membrane produce a sticky fluid called *mucus,* which coats the mucous membrane. Some of the cells also have hair-like structures on them (*cilia*), which beat rhythmically. The mucus lies on top of these cilia—a fact we shall talk about more later on.

The bronchioles also branch, finally ending in a cluster of little balloon-like structures called the *air sacs* or *alveoli.* There are about 300 *million* of these alveoli in the lungs. Thus, *one* trachea leads to *300 million alveoli;* clearly that involves a lot of branching! The alveoli have extremely thin walls. They also contain "elastic" tissue in their walls, making them behave much like tiny rubber balloons.

Step two: getting blood in and out

The system of blood tubes is similar in structure. It begins with one large tube (*main pulmonary artery*) that comes out of the right side of the heart (*right ventricle*). The *main* then splits into a right and left branch, one supplying each lung. Then each of these branches, like those in the bronchial system, divides many times into smaller and smaller *pulmonary arteries.* The smallest branches of this system also get a new name:

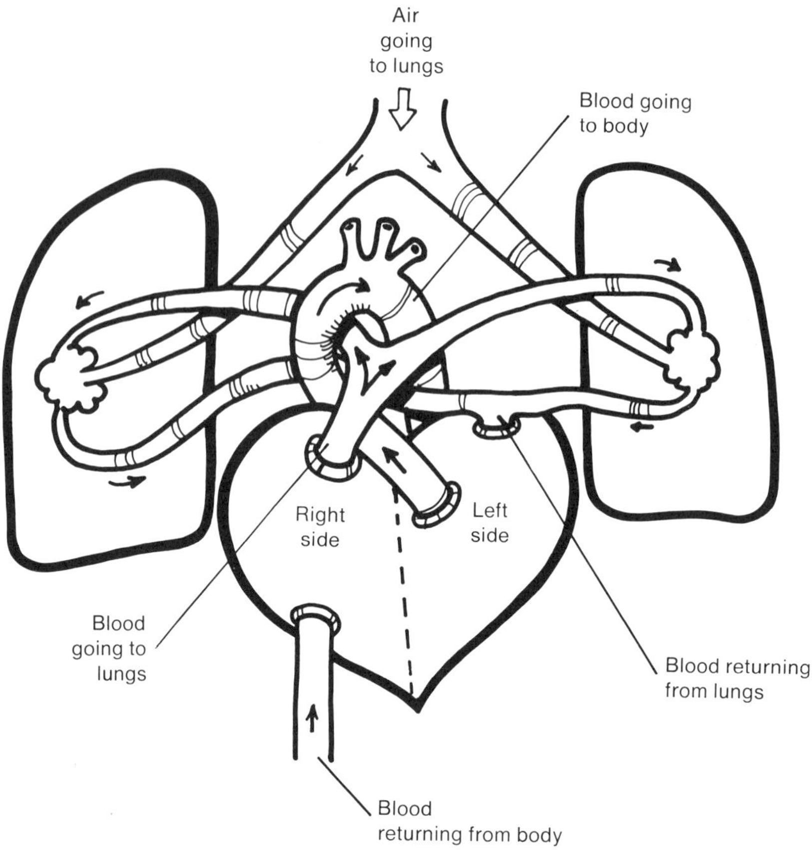

arterioles. The *arterioles* run along the walls of the *bronchioles.* Finally, the arterioles reach the *alveoli;* there they divide again into tiny vessels called *capillaries.* The capillaries are in the *walls* of the alveoli. Therefore, the blood in the capillaries is separated from the air in the alveoli only by the extremely thin, elastic walls of the alveoli. This is why it is normally so easy for oxygen to get into, and carbon dioxide out of, the blood. There are about one *billion* capillaries, more than three to each air sac.

Once the blood has passed through the capillaries (and taken up new oxygen and disposed of excess carbon dioxide), it goes to the left side of the heart (left atrium and ventricle). The left ventricle now pumps this "fresh" blood to the organs of the body through the *arteries.* Therefore, the arteries contain blood that has just come from the lungs. If the lungs are working properly, this blood contains a normal amount of oxygen and carbon dioxide; if they are not, the amount of oxygen and carbon dioxide may be abnormal—the oxygen decreased and the carbon dioxide increased. That is why blood is often taken from arteries and analyzed; these "arterial blood gas" values tell your doctor whether your lungs are doing their job.

There is often confusion in patients' minds about the "right side" and the "left side" of the heart. While both sides are in one package ("the heart") in your chest, you now know that the right heart pumps blood to the lungs; the left side receives this "fresh" blood and pumps it to the rest of the body. Therefore, the right heart can be directly affected by lung diseases. The left heart cannot. The blood in your arm or leg *veins* is returning to the right heart to be pumped to the lungs. The veins are bluish and do not pulsate. The blood in your arm or leg *arteries* contains blood that has just come from the lungs and is on its way to your organs (brain, kidney, muscles, and so on). The arteries usually cannot be seen, except as pulsations; but these pulsations are easily felt.

HOW THE "RESPIRATORY PUMP" WORKS

There are a few more things you should know about how the lungs work. For example, what makes air go into (*inspiration*) and out of (*expiration*) the lungs? The elastic lungs are contained within an airtight box, the chest or *thorax*. The cavity is sealed at its lower end by the *diaphragm*, a thin muscle that separates the chest from the abdomen ("stomach cavity"). It moves up and down like a piston. When it moves down (inspiration), the airtight thorax expands and a slight vacuum (negative pressure) is created. Air from the outside is therefore sucked into the lungs to overcome this vacuum. The elastic alveoli are stretched, like expanding balloons; then the diaphragm relaxes. The thorax becomes smaller, as do the elastic alveoli, which—again acting like balloons—expel the air from the lungs. For this system to work, it must be airtight so that a vacuum can be created during respiration. To assure this airtightness, the inner side of the chest wall and the outer side of the lungs are covered by a thin membrane (sheet of cells) called the *pleura*, which is moistened by a tiny amount of fluid so that the lungs slide smoothly as the thorax (chest wall) expands and contracts. Naturally, we are usually not aware of these things. Breathing normally goes on without our thinking about it; but as you know or will learn here, that is not the case if the lungs become abnormal. When the lungs become abnormal, muscles other than the diaphragm may be used to make the thorax larger and

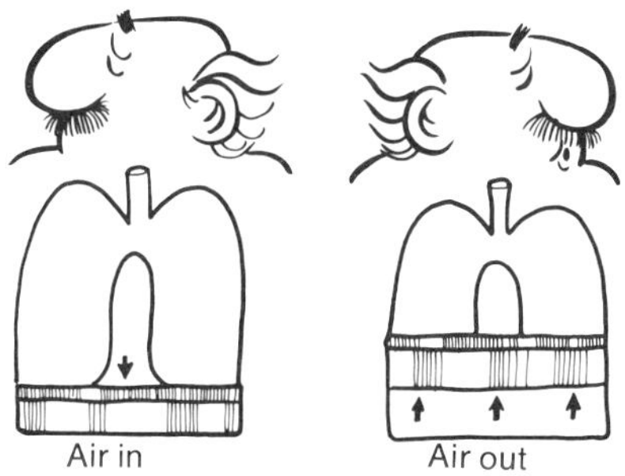

smaller. These are the *intercostal muscles* (which are between the ribs) and several muscles in the neck called *accessory muscles.* Usually, these muscles have little work to do during breathing; but in lung disease, they may have to do a great deal of work in breathing.

WHAT "CONTROLS" BREATHING?

There is another thing that most of us do not think about when we breathe. How do we know how *much* to breathe? What controls how deep and how fast we breathe? Actually, we have a complicated "control" system built into the body that works a lot like a thermostat for regulating a central heating/cooling system. The usual thermostat registers temperature and turns on or off the heater or air conditioner to keep the temperature where you want it. The "breathing thermostat" senses the oxygen and carbon dioxide in the blood. It turns on or off the breathing apparatus to keep oxygen and carbon dioxide levels in the blood at proper levels. If the oxygen level in the blood falls, or if the carbon dioxide rises, this "thermostat" makes you breathe harder (more quickly and deeper).

HOW THE LUNGS ARE PROTECTED

Finally, there are some things you should know about how the lungs *protect* themselves against impurities and other changes in the air we breathe. As you know, the air around us can be hot or cold or wet or dry, and can contain various irritating gases and particles. The lungs are rather delicate and work best when the air in them is moist, is at body temperature (37° C; 98.6° F), and is free of particles or irritating gases. Nature has designed several "protective" systems so that the lungs receive such air. The first of these systems is the *upper air passages*—the nose, the mouth, and the back of the mouth (oropharynx) where air entering the mouth or nose comes together. Above and around the nose and mouth are some "spaces" built into the skull called *sinuses.* These upper air passages and sinuses have two jobs: (1) to regulate the temperature and wetness of the air you breathe in and (2) to remove irritating particles and gases from this air. If the system works, air entering your windpipe will be at just the right temperature and wetness, and will be free of impurities. Thus, the upper air passages can warm or cool inhaled air, and can add or remove water from it; furthermore, irritant gases or particles are "trapped" in the mucus that coats these passages and are then removed by cough, sneeze, expectoration, or nose blowing.

If the upper air passages fail, or are unable, to do these things properly, air enters the lungs in less than perfect condition. The lungs themselves have several protection systems that then swing into action. The

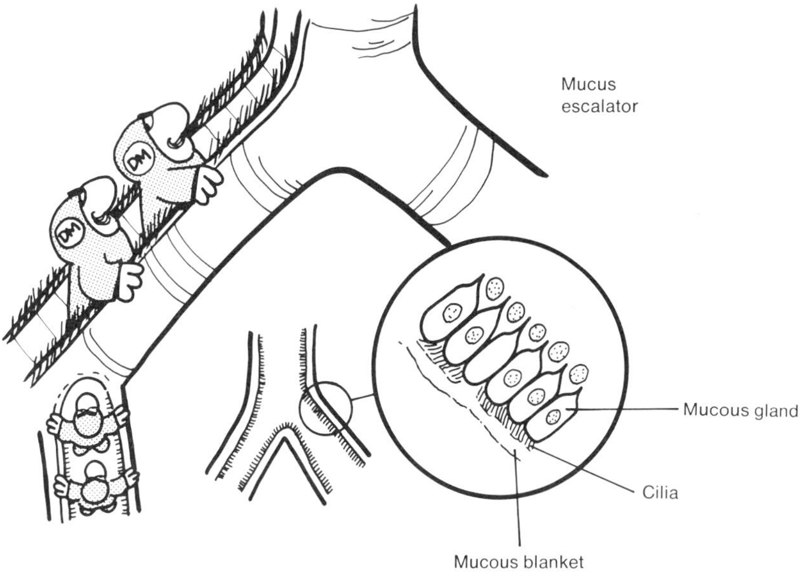

mucous membranes of the air tubes also are equipped to warm or cool air and to adjust its wetness. Particles or irritants also are "trapped" in the mucus that coats the bronchial tubes. After they are trapped, they can be coughed out or, more commonly, removed by a "mucus escalator" built into the lungs. There is a real "escalator" in the bronchial tree that consists of the mucous layer which is propelled from the small tubes to the windpipe by the cilia that beat toward the windpipe. This mucus is then either swallowed (without our being aware of it) or coughed out.

Of course, *cough* is another protection. Cough is produced by irritation of the bronchial tubes. This expels mucus much more rapidly than the "escalator." Cough also may alert us to the fact that we are inhaling irritating things and tells us to move away from them (if possible). Another "protection" is bronchial spasm. With severe irritation, the bronchial muscles contract, even in normal people. This is the body's way of trying to protect us from inhaling irritants (by clamping down the small bronchial tubes). The sensation is an unpleasant one, but again may alert us to an irritant exposure from which we should escape.

Finally, some irritating gases or particles may defy these elaborate protective systems and get to the air sacs. Even then, another defense system exists—a special kind of white blood cells called *macrophages.* These cells wander through the air sacs searching for debris—viruses, bacteria, particles that were inhaled. They engulf (suck up) such things, carry them off, and digest them. These cells cannot carry away all inhaled irritants. Some stay in the lungs and may cause future scarring or other problems.

This, then, is the way the normal lungs work, and how they are constructed. Knowing about these things should help you to understand how to take care of your lungs and how, when they are injured or abnormal, to help them to work better.

2 COPD—what does that mean?

COPD stands for *c*hronic *o*bstructive *p*ulmonary *d*isease. This term refers to a group of diseases that all share one common feature: difficulty in expelling air from the lungs. This is called *expiratory obstruction.*

In the past all persons with expiratory obstruction were lumped together and said to have COPD. However, we now know that several quite different diseases can cause expiratory obstruction. It is important to determine, in each patient, which cause or causes for expiratory obstruction exist, because the treatment for each is different. For example, medications that are helpful for one type of COPD are of little use in other types.

There are three diseases that cause COPD: chronic bronchitis, emphysema, and asthma.

CHRONIC BRONCHITIS

The problem in chronic bronchitis results from chronic inflammation and swelling of the cells lining the inside of the bronchi (air tubes). When inflamed, these cells produce excess quantities of mucus. The swelling of these cells narrows the air tubes, making breathing more difficult. The excess mucus narrows the tubes further and even blocks some completely. The irritation and excess mucus often cause chronic cough, in

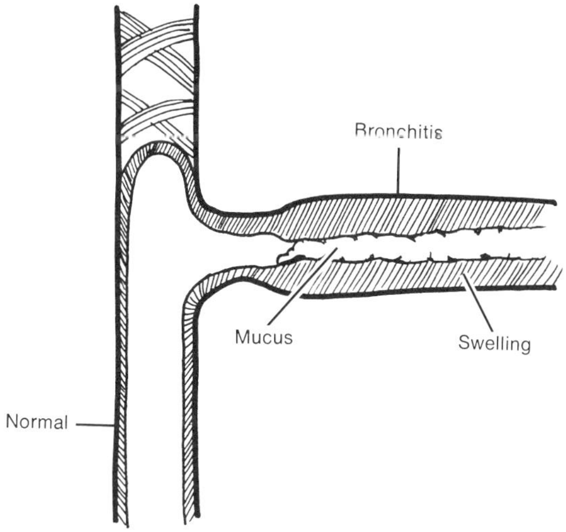

an attempt to expectorate the mucus. The lungs also become more easily infected because of these abnormalities. With repeated infections, lung damage may occur. Airways may become permanently dilated (bronchiectasis). Alveoli may become scarred (fibrosis). The narrowing of the bronchial tubes makes it more difficult for air to move in and out of them. If some tubes become blocked with mucus, the air sacs they supply cannot receive oxygen or get rid of carbon dioxide; they may, at least temporarily, collapse.

EMPHYSEMA

This refers to a disease in which the walls of the alveoli (air sacs) fracture (break). As these walls rupture, one air sac replaces two, four, or many more. The result is that there is a reduced number of air sacs (alveoli) and many of those that remain are enlarged. One large sac is less elastic than the many tiny sacs were. Thus, the patient with emphysema has lungs of reduced elasticity. To visualize the problems this causes, think of how a balloon works. You must blow (work) to fill it. But when you stop blowing, the balloon recoils (deflates) without your doing anything. The balloon's own elasticity causes it to expel the air. This is how normal alveoli work. You work (inspire) to inflate them with air. But when you relax, the lungs recoil (deflate) without effort on your part. Expiration (blowing air out of the lungs) is, therefore, a passive event. It just happens.

In emphysema the lungs and alveoli behave more like a paper bag. When you blow air into a paper bag, then stop blowing, what happens? Nothing. The bag stays full of air because it is nonelastic; it does not recoil. To empty the air from a paper bag, you must squeeze it out—and you must expend effort to push the air out. The patient with emphysema

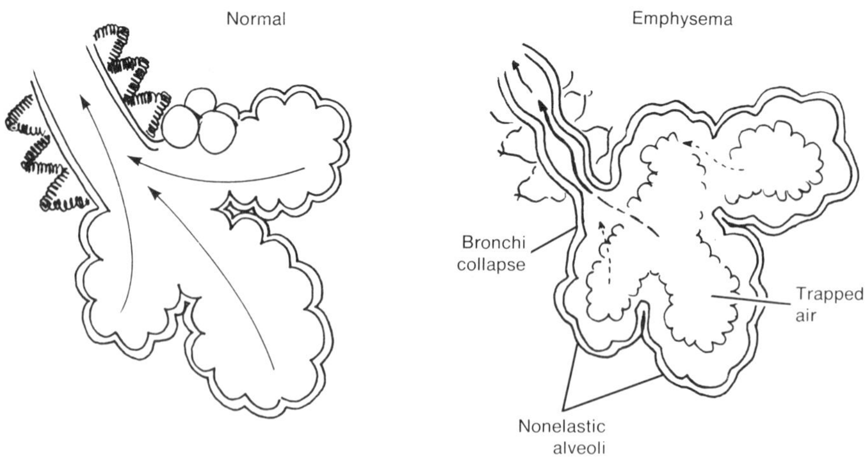

must do the same thing: expend energy during expiration to squeeze air out of the lungs.

Furthermore, this loss of lung elasticity affects the smaller bronchial tubes. To push air out of these less elastic lungs, a higher pressure must be developed inside the chest. This higher pressure tends to collapse the smaller bronchial tubes, making it even harder to empty air from the alveoli. This tendency to collapse also occurs with cough and makes it more difficult for the patient to cough up mucus. This collection of mucus, in turn, makes the lungs more susceptible to infection.

ASTHMA

The problem in asthma is that some irritant makes the muscles of the bronchial tubes go into spasm. This spasm narrows the bronchial tubes. Often, this same irritant causes the lining cells of the bronchial tubes to swell and increase their production of mucus (secretions). These changes further narrow and clog up the bronchial tubes. When these things happen, the patient notices sudden shortness of breath and sometimes wheezing.

There are several irritants that produce asthma. One is an *allergen,* that is, some material to which the patient is allergic. An allergy can show up as a rash, an upset stomach, or as bronchial spasm (asthma). Infection is another source of irritation; cold air, smog, and cigarette smoke are others.

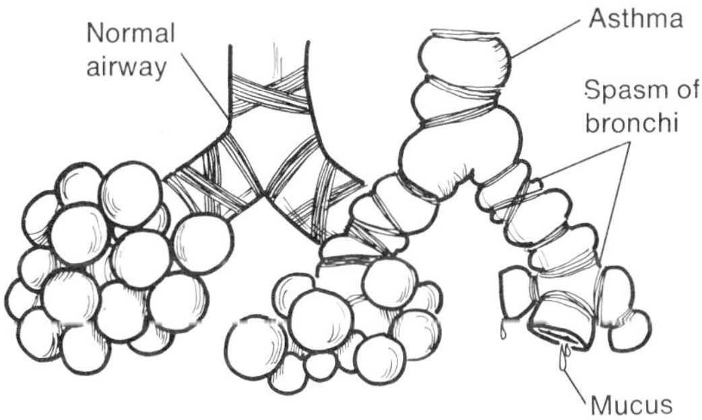

Many individuals with asthma have bronchial muscle that is more irritable than normal. Therefore, small amounts of inhaled irritants can cause bronchial spasm in them, but not in other people. This "hyper-irritability" of the bronchial tubes may run in families, that is, it may be inherited.

COPDs—A SUMMARY

Some patients have "pure" chronic bronchitis, emphysema, or asthma. Others have some combination of them. It is very important to know just what the problem is in a patient with COPD. Chest x-rays cannot make these distinctions. Pulmonary function tests can. These tests can tell your physician whether the symptoms are from emphysema, bronchitis, asthma—or some of each. Treatment depends on this information. Everyone with COPD has trouble breathing. But trouble breathing, like a pain in the chest, can mean many different things. The first step in dealing with your COPD is to find out what kind you have, because, as you now know, there is not one COPD; there are several types of chronic obstructive pulmonary diseases.

COPDs—HOW DO YOU GET THEM?

The causes of the chronic obstructive lung diseases have not been definitely determined. It is likely that the causes of emphysema, chronic bronchitis, and asthma are quite different. However, there are some features common to each. For example, heredity seems to play a role in the tendency to develop each disorder.

Air pollution, exposure to occupational dust and fumes, and lung infections make all forms of COPD worse. Allergy plays a role in some patients with asthma but not in emphysema or bronchitis. Most of these things cannot be controlled by the patient. But one factor *is* under the patient's control: cigarette smoking. Emphysema and chronic bronchitis rarely develop in nonsmokers; asthma is worsened by cigarette smoking.

COPDs—WHAT ARE THE SYMPTOMS?

Usually the first thing a patient with emphysema notices is shortness of breath on exertion (as when climbing stairs or walking quickly). Often this symptom is disregarded, and the individual feels it just means he or she is "out of shape." The first symptoms of chronic bronchitis are cough and mucus production. These symptoms are like a "chest cold" that hangs on week after week. Later, shortness of breath on exertion develops. The cough, mucus (sputum) production, and shortness of breath all may become suddenly worse if the patient develops the "flu" or some other type of lung infection.

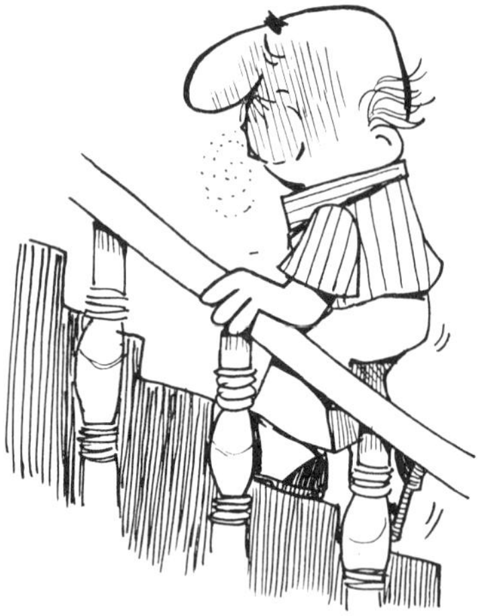

Asthma usually starts with rather sudden attacks of shortness of breath and wheezing. These attacks may come and go at first. Later on, mild wheezing and shortness of breath may be present all the time. The attacks may come at certain times of the year (particularly spring or fall), or after exposure to known allergens or irritants, or only during exercise, or with onset of a "cold." However, wheezing attacks also may appear without an obvious cause.

COPDs—HOW DO YOU KNOW YOU HAVE THEM?

The diagnosis of COPD involves many factors. The first step is for you to consult your doctor if you have any of the symptoms of COPD. The most common symptom is shortness of breath, particularly on exertion (walking up steps, carrying packages, hurrying during level walking). Patients first notice that they "can't keep up with" their spouses or friends. A chronic cough or wheezing may be other symptoms. Problems other than COPD can cause similar symptoms.

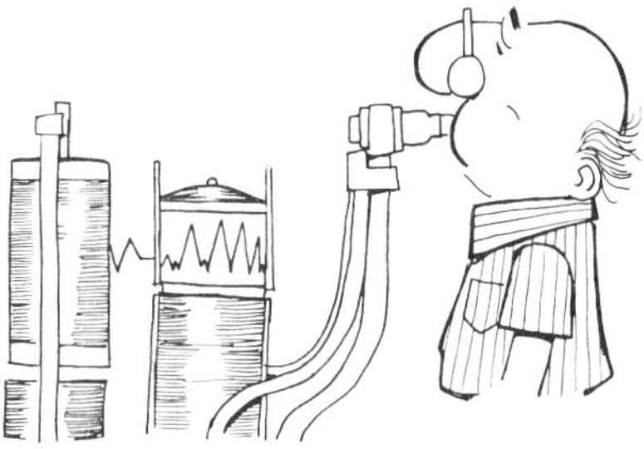

When you see your doctor, he will carry out a physical examination and other tests, such as pulmonary function tests, which may be necessary to determine whether you have a COPD—and, if so, what kind it is. The pulmonary function tests usually include breathing into one or more machines that measure how well your lungs are working. Also, a small blood sample may be taken from an artery while you rest and during exercise to determine how well the lungs are delivering oxygen

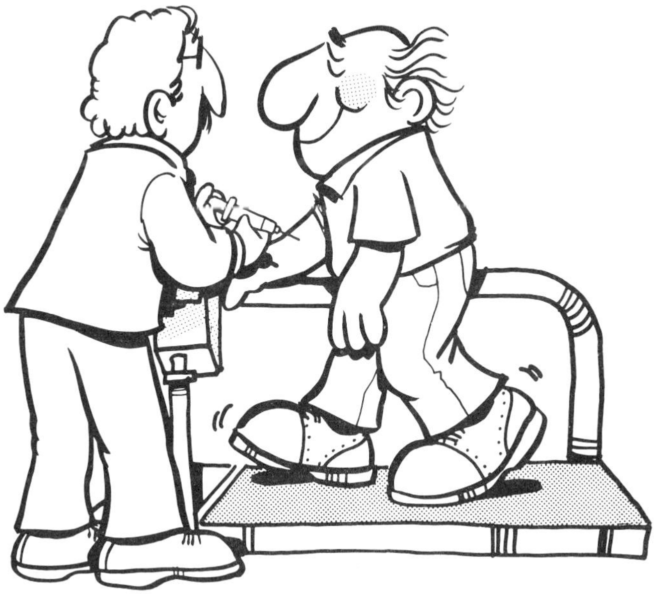

to the blood and removing carbon dioxide from it. A chest x-ray is taken to help in diagnosis. Based on this evaluation, your doctor can then develop a proper treatment plan designed for you.

COPDs—WHAT CAN BE DONE ABOUT THEM?

The most important factor in your treatment will be the relationship you have with your doctor. You must be willing to be frank and honest with him, and he must be the same with you. Some parts of your treatment will be his responsibility, such as prescribing drugs, treatments, tests, diets, and so on. A big responsibility is yours. You must take the medicines as ordered, do your treatments at home, practice proper breathing, eat correctly, and most important of all, quit smoking if you haven't already. The treatment of COPD is a cooperative venture. Each patient's disease is different.

Only your doctor knows which treatments and therapies are right for you. But only you know how you feel and how you respond to various treatments. Work with your doctor; ask him questions. The more you know about your disease, the better off you are. The more he knows about you, the better he can do his job.

The treatment of the COPDs may include some or all of the following:

- Medications
- Adequate diet
- Good hydration (fluid intake)
- Use of respiratory therapy
- Proper breathing techniques
- Maintenance of muscle tone
- Graded physical activity
- Bronchial drainage to remove excess mucus
- Prevention and treatment of infections
- Avoidance of allergens and/or irritants
- Weight control
- Use of supplemental oxygen in some cases

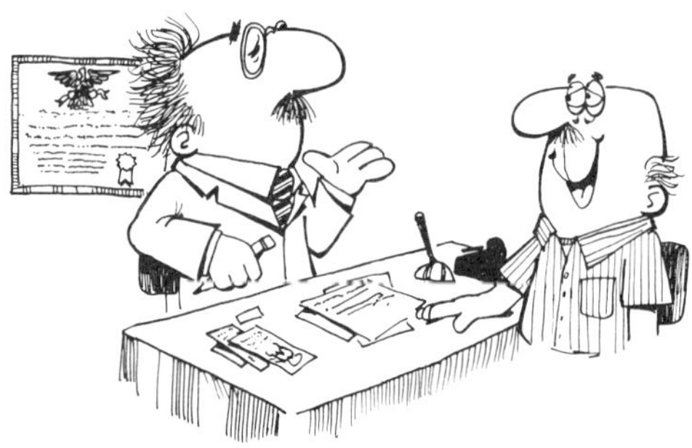

The precise nature of your type of COPD will determine the treatment prescribed. Sometimes very limited medication is all that is needed. Sometimes rather extensive treatment is required. The aims of treatment are to reverse the reversible, to preserve the function you have, and to teach you how to use the function you have more efficiently. These three aims can be achieved whether your problem is mild or severe.

COPD—WHAT IS YOUR RESPONSIBILITY?

Now that you have an understanding of what COPD means and the goals of treatment, it's time to add the most important ingredient—**you.** With enthusiasm, perseverance, and knowledge, you can play a big role in controlling your disease and alleviating some of your symptoms. The remainder of this manual is devoted to all aspects of treatment. After your doctor has outlined the various therapies he wants you to use, consult your manual for guidance and review.

3 Understanding your medications

A number of different medications are used to treat persons with the various types of COPD. Each medicine is designed to do a specific job to help the lungs function more effectively. Your doctor will determine which medications you need on the basis of your history, physical examination, breathing tests, and other laboratory studies.

All medicines are chemicals. They may come from plant sources or from animals. Some drugs are made entirely by man—these are "synthesized" drugs. Medicines are used for their beneficial effects, but they may also cause side effects: a medicine must enter the blood in order to reach the lungs; while on the way to the lungs it passes through many other organs and may exert other effects, called side effects. Most of the time these effects are well tolerated and may even disappear with time. You should be familiar with what your medicine is supposed to do and with its side effects.

Another important fact to remember is that each medicine has two names: a generic (chemical) name and a brand (company) name. The generic name is always the same for each drug, no matter which company manufactures it. The brand name for a drug is the property of the company that markets that drug. In some states it is possible for your pharmacist to substitute a less expensive generic brand drug for the more expensive branded product. Sometimes the practice may cause you some confusion and you may think you have received the incorrect prescription. If there are any questions because the pills look different to you, consult with your pharmacist. Besides providing you with medicines, many pharmacies provide other helpful services. For example, many pharmacists will maintain a complete record of all prescriptions you have received from any physician, dentist, or podiatrist. This "patient profile" can then be reviewed periodically by the pharmacist for drug interactions—a situation that occurs when two or more drugs taken at the same time work against each other. Ask your pharmacist or physician to explain this in more detail.

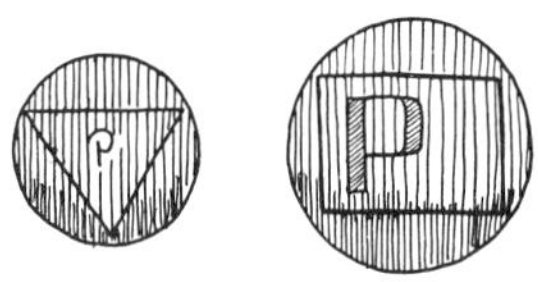

After each category of medication that follows, list, with the help of your physician or nurse, the names of the medications you take.

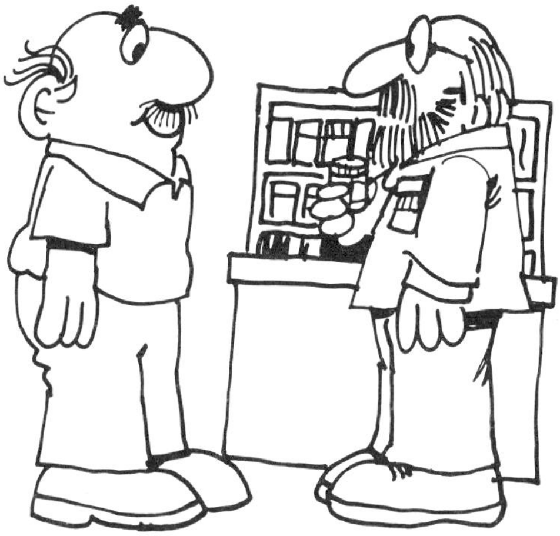

Bronchodilators. These drugs relax the muscles of the breathing tubes, thereby making them wider and allowing air to get in and out more easily. Bronchodilators can be taken as pills, liquids, or aerosol sprays (see Chapter 4). The most common of these drugs are theophylline (a xanthine), metaproterenol, and isoproterenol. Others are ephedrine and epinephrine (adrenaline). The xanthine drugs may cause an upset stomach and heartburn. Other of these drugs, depending on how they are taken (pill or spray) and on how much you use, can increase your heart rate and make you feel jittery or nervous.

______________________ ______________________

______________________ ______________________

Steroids. These drugs are all "relatives" of the hormone cortisol, which is normally produced by your body. These corticosteroids help to dilate the bronchial tubes, decrease the swelling of bronchial tube lining and also help to decrease lung inflammation. Steroids also have many potential side effects. They may make you feel very energetic and give you a sense of well-being. Other common side effects include weight gain, redistribution of fat, and easy bruising. The side effects depend upon the dose of the drug taken, how it is taken, and the length of time the therapy is continued. You must never discontinue oral steroids yourself or alter the dose without your physician's advice.

For many years, steroids could be taken only by pill or injection. Now certain special steroids (like Beclomethasone) have been developed that can be inhaled as an aerosol, directly into the lungs. They are absorbed very slowly and poorly into the blood. Therefore, they have beneficial effects on the lungs while causing very few side effects. These steroids must be taken on a *regular* schedule because they do not give immediate effects; rather, they prevent bronchospasm, so they are not to be used as you "need" them, but regularly, to prevent symptoms. Remember, these are potent medicines and must be taken only under the direction of your physician.

Cromolyn sodium. Cromolyn sodium is a medication used by patients who have asthma. Inhaled as a powder, it works only to prevent asthma and, to do so, must be taken regularly. It should never be used *during* an asthmatic attack, because it actually can make an attack worse.

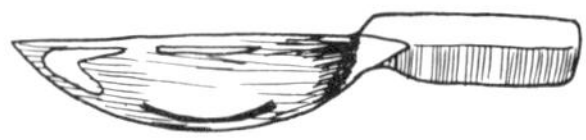

Expectorants. These drugs are intended to liquefy secretions and make them easier to cough up. Their value is debated, with no conclusive medical opinion as to whether they work or not. The most widely used expectorants are potassium iodide (SSKI) and glyceryl guaiacolate (GG). Potassium iodide can cause a rash and swelling of the salivary glands because of allergies to iodide.

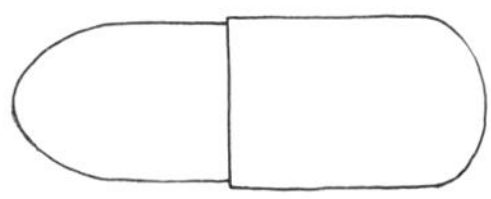

Antibiotics. These medications are used to fight bacterial infections. There are many different types that fight different bacteria. Some are given as pills or capsules, others by injection. Penicillin, sulfa drugs, and tetracycline are the generic names of the most commonly used drugs in this category. You should take these drugs in the exact dose and at the time specified by your doctor. He will tell you what side effects may occur. For example, an upset stomach or bowel problems are rather frequent with certain antibiotics. You must always finish the course of antibiotic therapy that your physician prescribes, even though you may feel better after only a few doses.

Diuretics (water pills). These medicines help rid your body of excess fluid. This fluid, called edema, usually shows up as swollen ankles and legs. There are a number of reasons why edema may develop in patients with lung disease. Diuretics need not be taken if only a little edema occurs in the ankles, but your doctor will make that decision. Overuse of diuretics can make you weak and should be avoided (see potassium supplements).

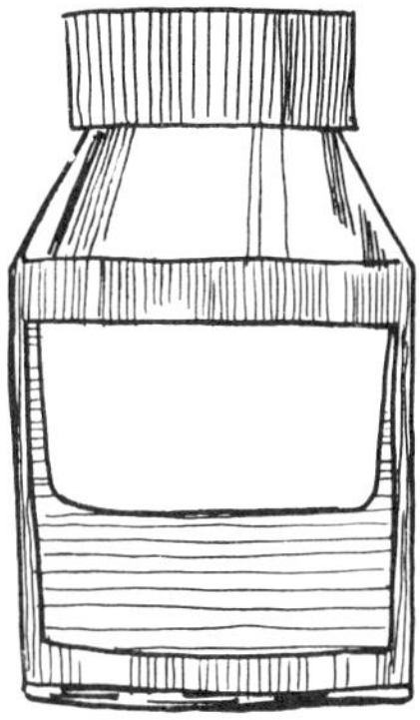

Digitalis. This is the generic, overall name for heart pills that strengthen the heart muscle. These drugs make the heart beat slower and with more force. Most patients with lung disease do not have heart problems that require digitalis, but some do. Digitalis drugs must be used carefully. The dose should never be changed without your doctor's order to do so.

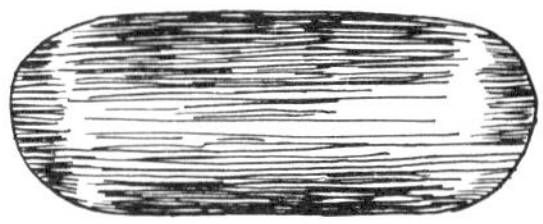

Potassium supplements. When diuretics are taken regularly, not only fluid but also potassium is lost. This may result in weakness and leg cramps. Potassium supplements are given to counteract these effects. Eating high-potassium foods is sometimes sufficient to replenish lost potassium (see Chapter 11).

Mood elevators. These medicines are designed to help you feel less depressed.

Tranquilizers and sedatives. These medicines are designed to calm or relax you and to help you sleep. These drugs can dangerously depress your breathing if taken in excess. The dose should, therefore, never be increased without consulting your doctor—no matter how nervous or tense you are. Such symptoms (insomnia, irritability) may mean that your lungs are not working properly and that sedatives and tranquilizers should be decreased, not increased. Your physician knows which medicines are best for you.

______________________ ______________________

______________________ ______________________

Flu and pneumonia vaccines. These help you to fight off serious viral (flu) infections and certain other (pneumococcal) infections. These are usually given in the fall before the start of the flu season.

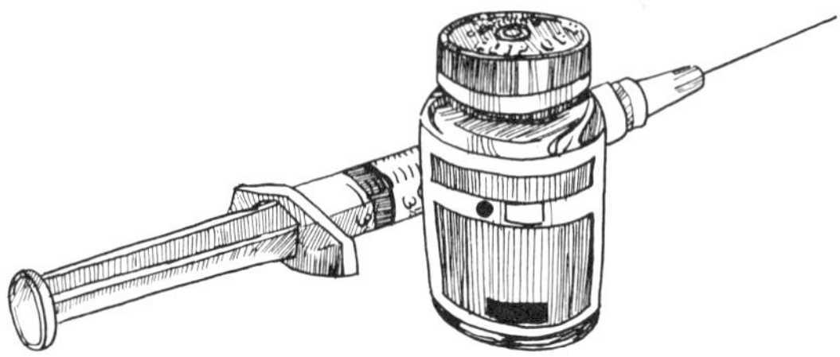

Oxygen. Sometimes patients with lung disease cannot transfer enough oxygen from the alveoli to the blood; therefore the amount of oxygen in the blood falls below normal levels. Such a low blood oxygen level impairs the body's engine (see Chapter 1). People with perfectly normal lungs have the same problem at high altitudes (or when they become astronauts and want to walk around on the moon, where the atmosphere contains no oxygen!). Whatever the reason for the oxygen lack, the treatment is the same: take a drug that overcomes the deficiency. In the case of oxygen deficit, that "drug" is oxygen.

Like all drugs, oxygen must be prescribed by your doctor and used with great care. The drugs you take for your respiratory problem are ordered by your doctor in a specific *amount*, at specific *times*, to be taken by a specific *route*. For example, aminophylline (drug), 250 mg. (dose), four times a day (times), by mouth (route). Likewise, oxygen is prescribed by your doctor in the same manner: oxygen (drug), 2 liters/minute (dose), during exercise (time), by nasal cannula (route). Your doctor decides upon the appropriate dose based on blood oxygen measurements taken at rest and while exercising. As with other drugs, the dosage of oxygen must not be increased or decreased without the doctor's advice. Turning the liter flow above the prescribed dose may cause serious complications—too much oxygen can injure your lungs and can make your breathing worse. (See Chapter 4 for more information on the use of oxygen.)

• • •

Remember that millions of dollars each year are spent on medicines. You can help make the most of your medicine dollar by taking your medications as prescribed by your physician. Each person should receive those medicines that are best for him or her. Those which are good for **you** may not necessarily be good for your **friend** or **relative!**

4 Breathing paraphernalia

Most patients with COPD sooner or later are treated with some type of respiratory therapy equipment or hear about such equipment from others. Often, it is first used during a hospitalization and patients are not certain why it was used or whether it might be useful at home.

Many ingenious kinds of respiratory therapy equipment have been developed for use by patients with COPD. The equipment varies widely in complexity, cost, and usefulness. The device that gave you so much relief in the hospital may present many problems for you at home and may not be of value there. Often you can do things yourself that will help your breathing more than any machine! There is no substitute for being informed about your disease.

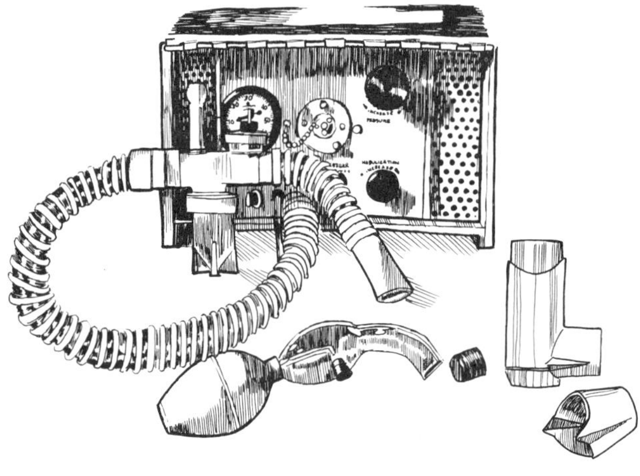

If you do need equipment at home, the simplest device that will do the job is the best choice. **Remember: The more complex the equipment, the bigger your commitment is for its use, care, and maintenance.** To achieve maximum benefits you should clearly understand the purpose and correct usage of the equipment prescribed for you.

Also, be aware that cost is not a good measure of the value of a device. Inexpensive devices are often as effective as costly ones. Fancy dials and gadgets are no indication that you are getting "the best."

Your doctor should be familiar with these devices. He will indicate whether you need them, and which bests suits your condition.

The most frequently used devices for home care can be conveniently listed under two categories—oxygen therapy and aerosol therapy. We shall describe the equipment associated with the delivery of oxygen as *oxygen therapy equipment* and the devices which produce visible mist for inhalation as *aerosol therapy equipment.* You may also receive a combination of these treatments.

OXYGEN THERAPY

What is oxygen? It is an element, a drug, and a gas. Every cell in the body needs energy to function. Cells get their energy from a combination of the food we eat, plus oxygen. This energy enables us to use our muscles to breathe, to perform work, and to carry out all bodily functions.

The process by which the body takes in oxygen and eliminates carbon dioxide is called gas exchange (see Chapter 1). If gas exchange does not occur normally, then the oxygen in your blood will be decreased. This is determined by an arterial blood test. If necessary, your doctor will prescribe supplemental oxygen for you (see Chapter 3).

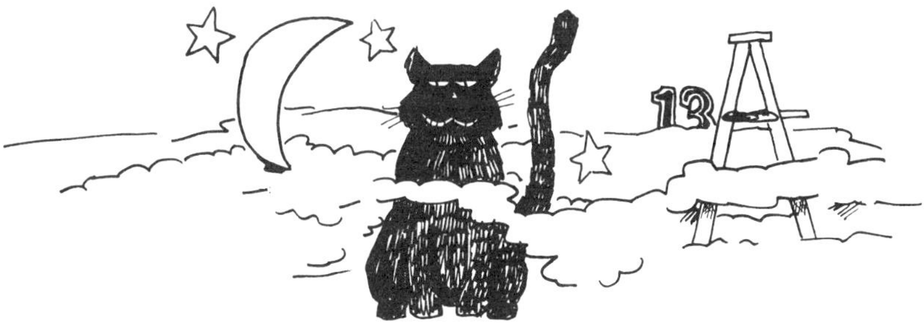

MYTHS AND TRUTHS ABOUT OXYGEN

Myth: Oxygen is addicting. Once you start it, you will have to use it forever.
Truth: *Oxygen is not addicting.* You need use it only when your own lungs cannot supply enough. When you no longer need it, you can stop it.

Myth: If a little oxygen is good, a lot of oxygen is better.
Truth: *Oxygen is a drug.* Use it only as instructed. Like any drug, too much can be injurious.

Myth: Shortness of breath means lack of oxygen, so if you become short of breath, you should take oxygen.
Truth: *Shortness of breath is not always associated with oxygen lack.* If oxygen lack is not the cause, taking oxygen will do no good. Your doctor can test to see whether you need oxygen by taking blood from an artery and measuring the amount of oxygen (arterial blood gas).

Myth: People who need to use oxygen must be confined to their homes and can't do anything.

Truth: *People who use oxygen can lead a normal life.* There are several types of portable oxygen systems available. With good prior planning, you can be active and mobile. Using portable oxygen is not that different from using a hearing aid or glasses—it's just bulkier.

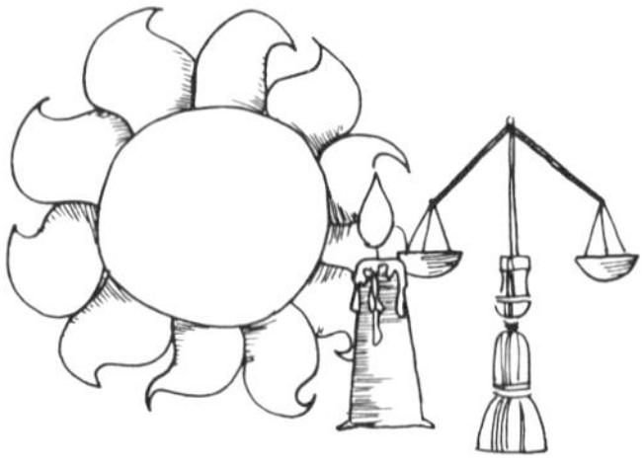

YOU AND O_2 AT HOME

Oxygen makes up 21% of the air around us. This oxygen can be extracted from the air by a very special industrial process, which yields 100% oxygen that has been purified and dehumidified. Now the oxygen is ready for packaging and home deliveries.

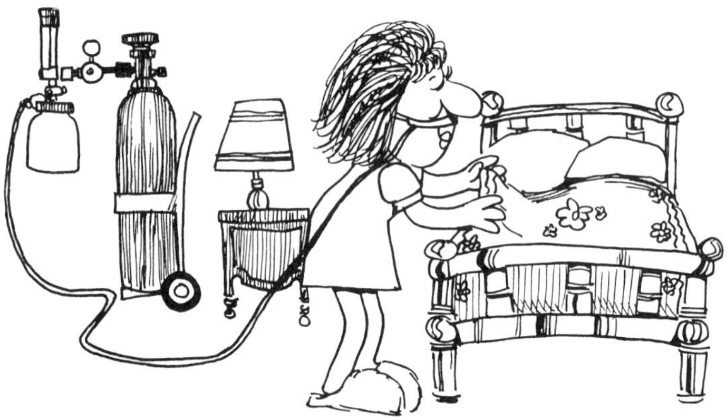

Today there are a wide variety of systems available for home use. Oxygen can be purchased as compressed gas or as a liquid. You can also purchase or rent electrical devices that generate oxygen from room air. Some oxygen sources are portable; some are not. The selection of oxygen sources to choose from is broader than ever before and is improving yearly.

When deciding which one will suit your needs, consider these points:

1. Cost—Will your medical insurance reimburse you for this particular oxygen system?
2. Life-style—Are you sedentary or active?
3. Content—Will the portable unit you select provide you with enough oxygen for doctor's appointments, shopping trips, and social activities?

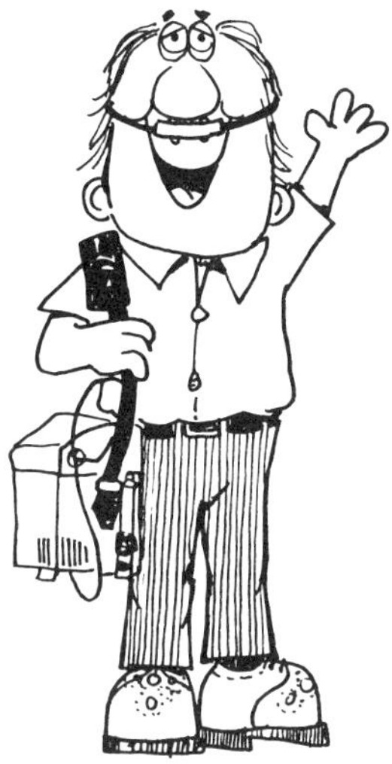

Safety and storage

Oxygen is a relatively safe gas, but because it supports combustion, it must be handled with caution. Oxygen itself does not burn, but it aids in igniting combustible materials. For example, any spark or open flame expands markedly like a "flashfire." Also, oxygen in tanks is under high pressure; therefore, if the top of the tank is knocked loose, the tank can "take off" like a rocket. Liquid oxygen is very cold, and touching the "steam" that may escape can burn you.

Remember:

1. The room in which oxygen is stored should be dry, cool, and well ventilated; keep oxygen away from heat, flame, and spark sources.
2. Be certain that the oxygen is fastened securely. This will prevent it from being knocked over.
3. Avoid inhaling irritating debris that may accumulate at the bottom of cylinders by always changing them when the pressure regulator reads 500 psi (pounds per square inch).
4. Never permit grease, oil, or any other potentially combustible substance to come into contact with oxygen delivery equipment.
5. Smoking is not permitted within 10 feet of a source from which oxygen is being administered. Also, there must be at least 10 feet between the oxygen source and any open flame or possible source of electrical sparks.

Think ahead

When your oxygen tank is first delivered, determine how many hours each tank will last at your prescribed liter flow. Keep enough on hand so that deliveries can be made on a regular schedule and you won't run out at night or during a weekend. When your oxygen is delivered, have the technician explain the formula for determining when you should order a refill.

Oxygen regulator

A compressed gas cylinder has a regulator and flowmeter attached to it. A *regulator* is a device that reduces the high pressure of the oxygen as it leaves the cylinder. The regulator also tells you how much oxygen is in the cylinder: a full tank of oxygen usually contains 2200 psi pressure. As you use oxygen, the pressure reading of the cylinder will decrease. If you use liquid oxygen, the contents are determined by weighing the container with a scale.

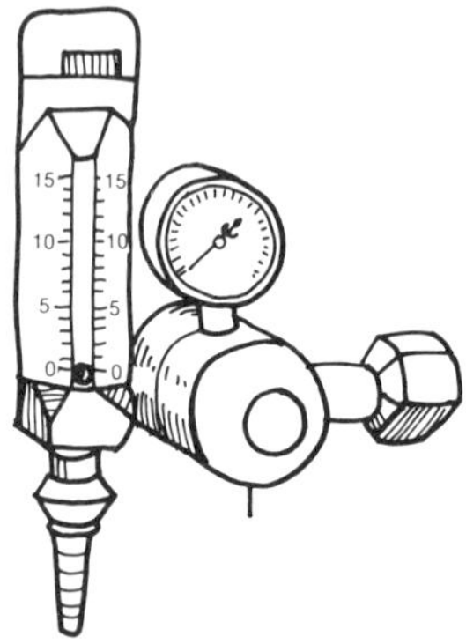

The *flowmeter* is a measuring device or dial; it is part of the oxygen regulator or is attached to your liquid oxygen container or concentrator. Never use oxygen without a flow control. The flowmeter regulates how much oxygen is delivered to you in liters per minute (see Chapter 3). This is determined and prescribed for you by your doctor.

Oxygen concentrator

This is a new type of system for oxygen delivery that is useful for some patients. This device is an electrical unit that looks like a nightstand or endtable. The concentrator "makes its own oxygen" by remov-

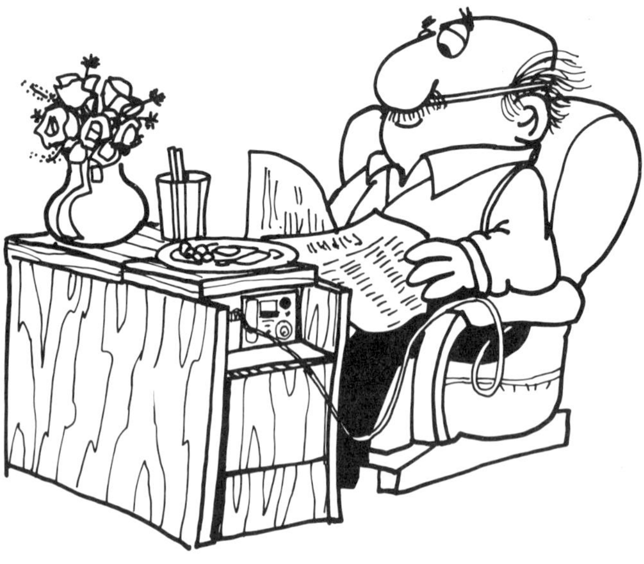

ing the oxygen molecules from room air. There are several advantages to using this method of oxygen therapy:

1. It may be less expensive.
2. It does not require refilling or replacement of cylinders.
3. It is easier to manage.
4. It has an attractive appearance.

Humidifier

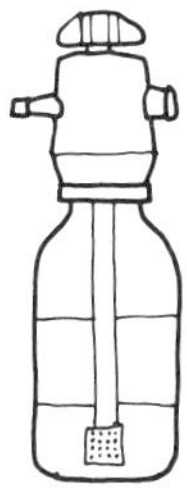

A humidifier is a bottle or jar filled with water and attached to an oxygen flowmeter. The purpose of the humidifier is to replace water vapor that has been removed from oxygen during the process of manufacturing.

Nasal cannula or venturi mask

These are the two preferred appliances for oxygen delivery. The nasal cannula is most often the choice for people using oxygen at home.

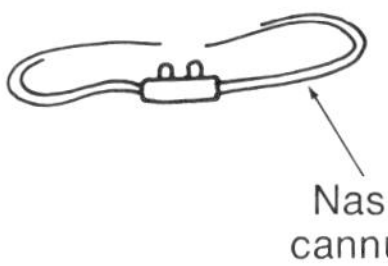

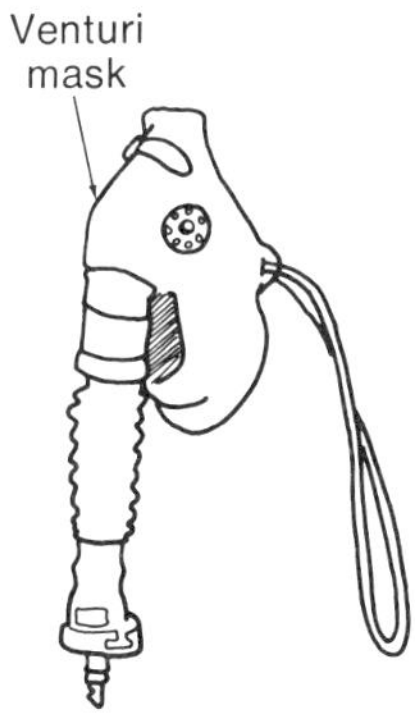

AEROSOL THERAPY

The respiratory therapy devices discussed here are those associated with aerosol or "mist" therapy. This treatment modality involves the inhalation of medications and/or water directly into the air passages of the lungs. Inhaling medications is a relatively fast and reliable method for symptom relief. Chest congestion with thick secretions and an ineffective cough can often be relieved with the inhalation of medications and water.

Metered dose device (MDD)

This is a very simple, easy-to-handle, and convenient mode for inhalation of medications. It consists of a small cartridge containing various types of medicine, chiefly bronchodilators or steroids (see Chapter 3), and a mouthpiece for dispensing the drug. The advantage of this type of aerosol therapy is its portability and minimal care, as well as its quick action.

INSTRUCTIONS FOR METERED DOSE DEVICE (MDD)

1. Assemble MDD for use.
2. Exhale *completely* through pursed lips. (See Chapter 5.)
3. Place open end of mouthpiece into your mouth past front teeth, as shown in figure at right.

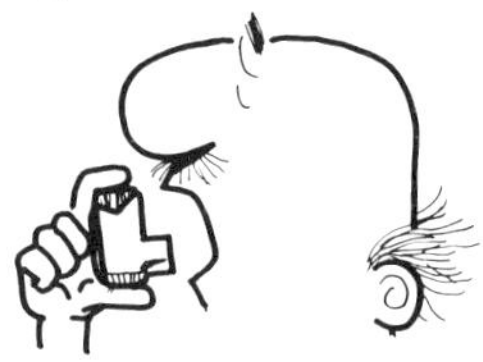

4. *Do not* close lips—this allows more air to be inhaled through the mouth to aid in carrying the medication deeper into air passages.
5. While taking a slow deep breath, press down firmly on cartridge to release medication.
6. Hold your breath a few seconds to allow medication to settle on the surface of your airways. (This will prevent you from exhaling the medication and aid in obtaining relief.)
7. Exhale slowly, using pursed lips.
8. Repeat only as prescribed; rest a few moments before using again.
9. Keep MDD clean and free from dirt, lint, and so on by placing it in a clean plastic bag.
10. Wash and disinfect plastic mouthpiece dispenser regularly.
11. Periodically check the amount of medication in your MDD so that you may obtain refills ahead of time. An easy way to estimate how much medication is left inside is to place the cartridge in a container of water and observe its position as it floats.

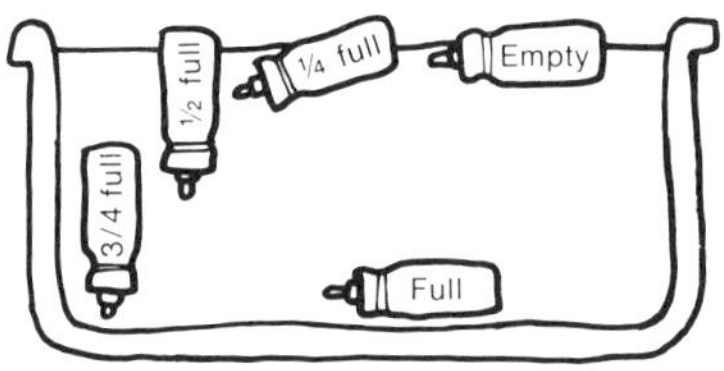

Note: Do not overuse. **Use only as directed** by your doctor.

Nebulizers—the big, the small, and the ultrasonic

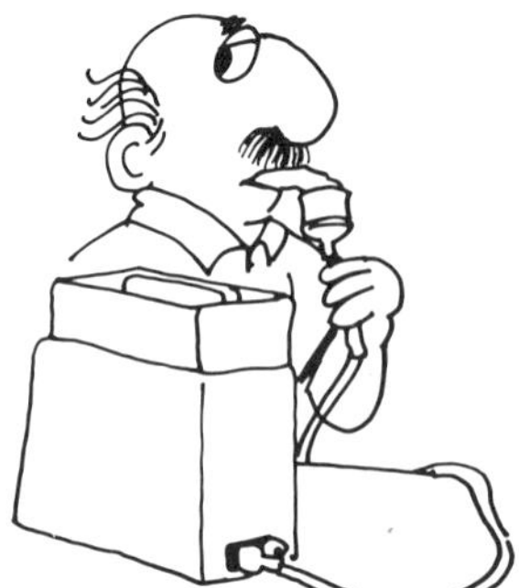

A nebulizer is a device that is designed to mechanically produce a mist or fog from a liquid; it can be powered either by pressurized air, by oxygen, or by an electrical source.

A very popular set-up for aerosol therapy at home is the "mini-neb" and air compressor. This system is compact, is simple to operate, and requires little maintenance. It is used primarily to deliver medications or moisture for short periods of time, intermittently throughout the day. The maximum capacity of a small nebulizer is approximately 15 ml (1 tablespoon).

Nebulizers are also available for continuous use. These units have a much larger capacity (250 to 500 ml). This is the preferred method of delivering moisture to the air passages of individuals with a tracheostomy (temporary or permanent tube placed in the trachea via an opening at the base of the neck).

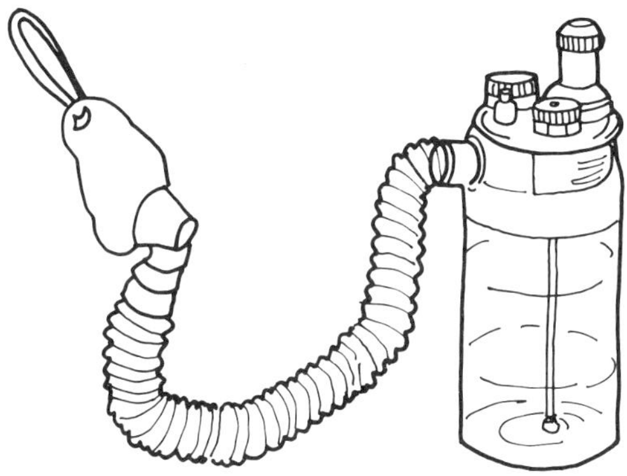

The ultrasonic nebulizer is a very effective nebulizer that operates from an electrical source. Unlike the above-mentioned nebulizers, this unit transforms electrical energy into vibrations, which are then transferred to a liquid. Vibration of the liquid results in a fine, dense, cool mist. This device is more expensive than conventional jet nebulizers and should be considered for home use only when other aerosol devices do not yield the desired results.

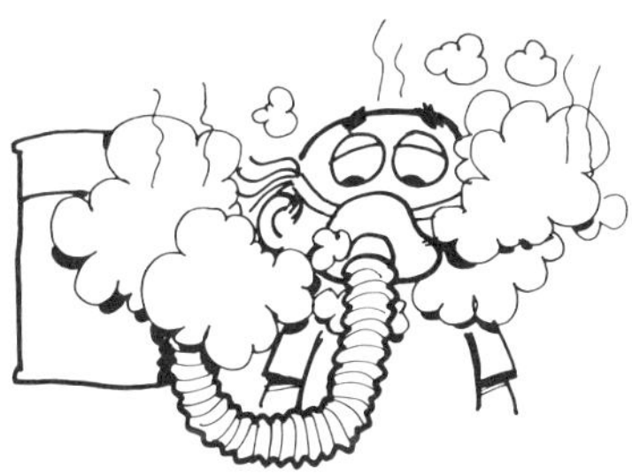

Everything you ever wanted to know about aerosol therapy but were afraid to ask and should know

1. The name of the equipment you are using and its parts.
2. How often you should take it (for example, twice a day), and for how long (for example, 20 minutes).
3. What solutions to put in the nebulizer.
4. How to prepare, store, and measure the solutions you are using.
5. What parts of the nebulizer unit should be removed for cleaning.
6. How to clean and disinfect your nebulizer (must be done every 24 hours).

7. How to troubleshoot minor malfunctions.
8. **Most important:** the correct breathing pattern to use while taking aerosol therapy. We recommend slow, deep breathing and a slight pause after full inspiration to allow the liquid particles to settle in the lungs.

How to prepare sterilized water or normal saline for home use

Here are instructions for making your own solutions for inhalation. Many times it will be easier and less expensive for you to prepare them. Remember that bacteria can grow in your solutions unless you are extremely careful! Please follow these instructions exactly as they are written.

1. You need a jar with a lid that fits snugly. A small jam jar or juice bottle will do.
2. Thoroughly wash this jar and its lid in detergent; rinse.
3. Place the jar and its lid in a pan and fill with tap water so that the jar is completely submerged. Place a lid on the pan and gently boil the jar for 15 minutes to sterilize it.
4. After you have boiled the jar, pour the tap water out of the pan. (Use the pan lid to prevent the sterilized jar from falling out.)
5. After the jar and lid have cooled, removed them from the pan. Place them upright on a clean counter. **Do not** let anything "unsterile" touch the insides of the jar or lid. **Do not** dry them with a towel or place them upside down to drain.
6. Resterilize the jar and lid *at least* once each week.
7. Pour distilled water (twice the desired amount) into the clean pan used to boil the jar. If preparing normal saline (salt water), add 1/4 teaspoon of salt to every 2 cups of distilled water.
8. Boil gently for 15 minutes. You will have about half the water you started with. Let the water cool and then pour it into the "sterile" jar; cover with lid.
9. Store this in the refrigerator; discard any unused solutions at least once a week.
10. To remove any solution from the jar, pour it directly into your nebulizer. Never place an "unsterilized" eyedropper, teaspoon, or other measuring device into the solution in the jar. Do not pour any extra solution back into the jar once it has been removed—discard it.

Intermittent positive pressure breathing (IPPB)

Intermittent positive pressure breathing (IPPB) must be prescribed by your doctor, the only one who can determine if you *need* this type of treatment. IPPB is a highly specialized method of delivering aerosol therapy to the lungs. The medication and/or moisture is carried from the machine's nebulizer into your lungs by the flow of *air* under *pressure.* In other words, this device assists you in breathing and can help you take a deeper breath. This apparatus includes a variety of attachments and tubes and is more complicated than any of the other treatment modalities.

If IPPB is indicated, your doctor's prescription should contain the following:

Frequency of treatments (twice a day)
Duration of treatment (15 minutes)
Type of medication and amount to use (for example, bronchodilator medicine and normal saline)
Pressure setting (15 cm H_2O pressure)

Your doctor or a therapist will instruct you in the use and care of your machine. **Be certain that you thoroughly understand the use and precautions of IPPB before administering at home.**

CHECKPOINTS BEFORE TAKING EACH TREATMENT

1. Be sure tubing and accessories are clean and dry.
2. Be sure the equipment set-up is properly connected to your machine.
3. Place the correct dose of medication in the nebulizer cup:
   a. Use a clean eyedropper or syringe.
   b. Cap all medication bottles after use.
   c. Pour saline or water directly into nebulizer cup.
   d. After opening, store medication bottles in refrigerator.
4. Set pressure knob according to your prescription.
5. Turn machine on and check for mist production at the mouthpiece.

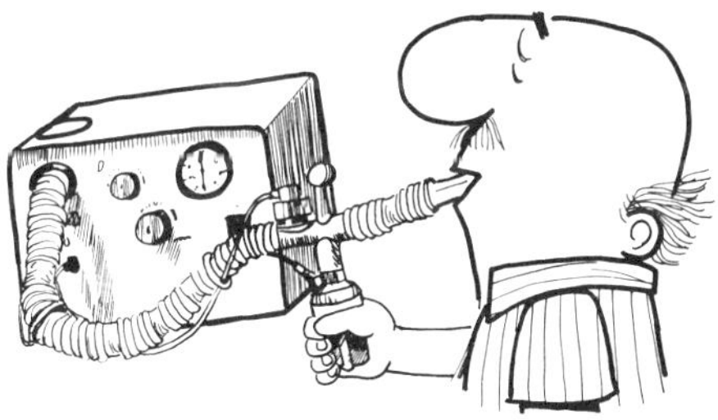

TAKING YOUR IPPB TREATMENT

1. Sit in an upright position. Relax.
2. Set the kitchen timer or check your watch before starting.
3. Be sure the nebulizer is in an upright position and the tubes are not bent or kinked.
4. Place mouthpiece between your teeth and bite gently, keeping your

lips tight around it so air does not escape. (A nose clip may be needed.)
5. Begin inspiration; this first part of breathing-in activates (turns on) the positive pressure machine. Then take a slow deep breath, letting the air from the machine fill your lungs. (The machine will cycle off when the pressure your doctor has ordered is reached.) Hold your breath for 2 seconds before exhaling. Then exhale slowly. Always remember to breathe *very slowly* and *exhale completely.* Rest between breaths on the machine.
6. IPPB treatments help bring up sputum. Don't hesitate to stop your treatment to cough.
7. Your mouth may become dry during or after a treatment. You may stop your treatment for a drink of water.

AFTER YOUR TREATMENT

1. After each treatment, disassemble and wash, then rinse the nebulizer and mouthpiece. Shake off excess water, and place these parts on a clean paper towel. Cover with another paper towel until next treatment.
2. After the last treatment of the day, follow instructions on your cleaning sheet for daily cleaning procedure.

NOTE: If you have any discomfort or strange sensations during or after IPPB treatments, notify your doctor.

CARE AND CLEANING OF YOUR RESPIRATORY EQUIPMENT

You must take proper care of all equipment that delivers mists or medications into your lungs. If your equipment is contaminated with bacteria, even your own bacteria, you can reinfect yourself and put an extra strain on your lungs and heart. Be sure you clearly understand what equipment parts need to be washed and disinfected. Ask your doctor, therapist, or equipment rental company to explain an effective technique. (We recommend daily cleaning for any mist-producing equipment.)

The following instructions offer an approach that is simple and inexpensive. **All equipment you use must be cleaned daily.**

Supplies needed

Liquid detergent (such as Joy)
White vinegar
Soft brush
Two basins or buckets (Do not use sink.)

1. Basin 1 should contain detergent water (discard daily).

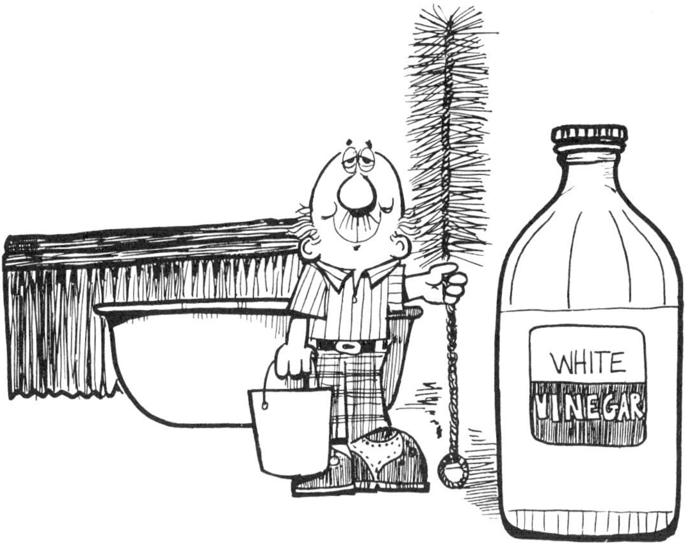

2. Basin 2 should hold one part vinegar to one part water (discard every other day; cover between use).

The routine for cleaning

1. Remove all washable parts of equipment and disassemble.
2. Wash in warm soapy water (basin 1). Scrub all parts gently with brush. Get into all crevices to remove medications, secretions, or any foreign material.
3. Rinse thoroughly under tap water.
4. Soak equipment in vinegar solution (basin 2) for a minimum of *30 minutes* (to kill bacteria). Be sure hollow parts are filled with solution and equipment is completely submerged.
5. Rinse completely under hot tap water; be careful not to touch the sink with your equipment.
6. Air-dry your equipment by:
   a. Shaking or swinging excess water out of tubing and hard-to-dry areas of accessories
   b. Hanging tubing to allow to drip dry completely
   c. Placing all other pieces of equipment on clean paper towels and covering with paper towels

Remember

1. Discard detergent solution (basin 1) daily.
2. Vinegar solution (basin 2) should be

covered and can be kept for 2 days, but no longer. Store in a clean area.

3. Wipe down all surfaces of the machine with a clean damp cloth daily. Then cover and store in a clean area between treatments.
4. Use scrub brush and basins only for equipment cleaning.
5. Store *dry* tubing and accessories in unused sealed plastic bags.
6. Have two complete sets of washable equipment so you always have a clean, dry set-up available for use the following day.

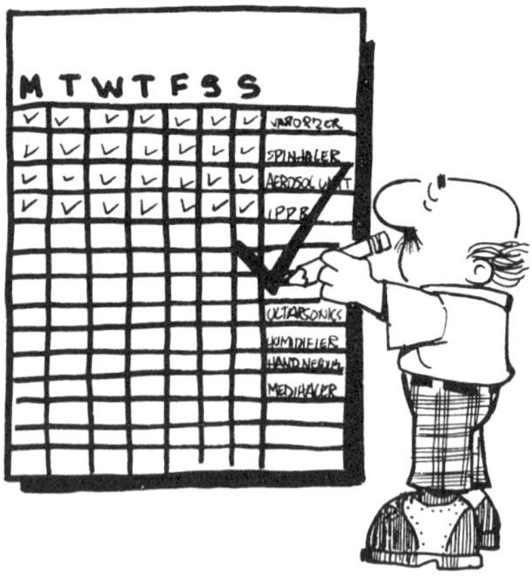

7. Hair dryers or blowers are *not* to be used to dry equipment.

All equipment must be washed as stated every 24 hours!

5 The art of better breathing and coughing

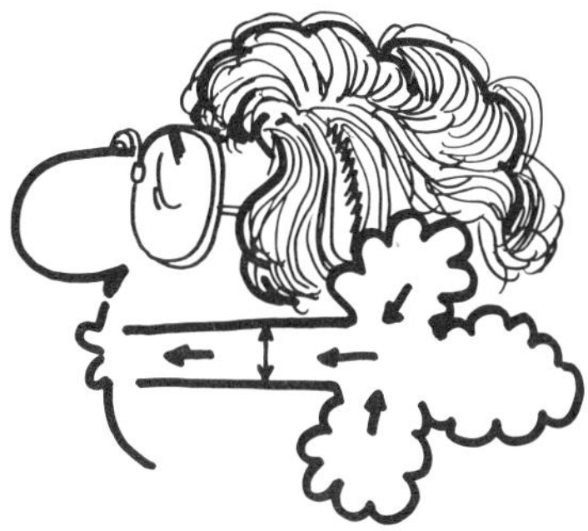

BREATHING EXERCISES

Pursed lip breathing

The purpose of this breathing technique is to aid you in removing trapped air from your lungs. In COPD, airways can collapse when you exhale and trap stale air in the air sacs. When this happens, there is not enough room for you to breathe in fresh air. Pursed lip breathing provides a resistance to exhaled air at the mouth level and maintains a higher pressure in the airways. This keeps the airways open longer so that more air can get out.

1. Inhale through your nose with your mouth closed.
2. Exhale through your mouth with your lips pursed. (Pursed lips means having your lips in a whistling or kissing position.)
3. Make your exhalation at least twice as long as your inhalation (for example, 2 seconds in, 4 seconds out).

You may want to spend more time breathing out (for example, 2 seconds in, 6 seconds out). Don't force air out to the point of discomfort.

Pursed lip breathing is a basic technique used with all other breathing exercises. When you become short of breath, it should be practiced along with diaphragmatic breathing. Learn it first and learn it well.

Diaphragmatic breathing

Normal movement of the diaphragm

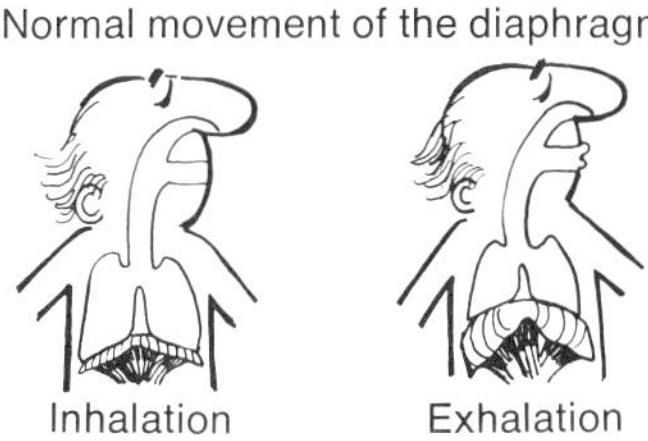

The purpose of this exercise is to reactivate and strengthen the diaphragm. Normally the diaphragm does about 80% of the work of breathing. In COPD the diaphragm flattens and the upper chest muscles try to take over. These muscles require more oxygen to do the diaphragm's job. To locate your diaphragm, place your flat hand on the center of your stomach at the base of the breast bone—then sniff. You will feel your diaphragm move.

EXERCISE 1—FRONT EXPANSION

Assume a comfortable position as indicated in the picture.

1. Place one hand in the center of your stomach at the base of your breastbone—this hand will detect the movement of your diaphragm.
2. Place your other hand on your upper chest—this hand will detect the movement of your accessory muscles.
3. Exhale slowly through pursed lips while drawing your stomach muscles inward (Figure A).
4. Inhale slowly through the nose—your stomach should expand outward (Figure B). The hand over the diaphragm should feel the most movement.
5. Rest.

A

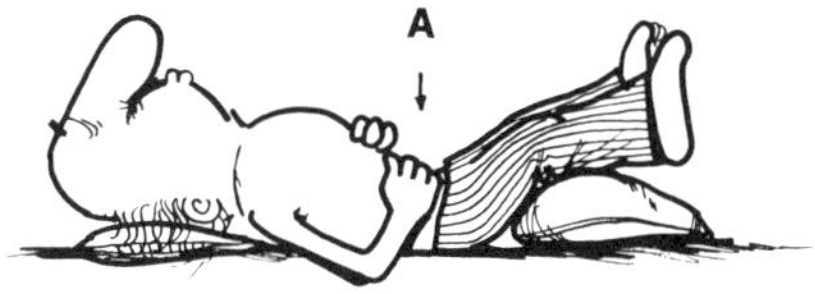

B

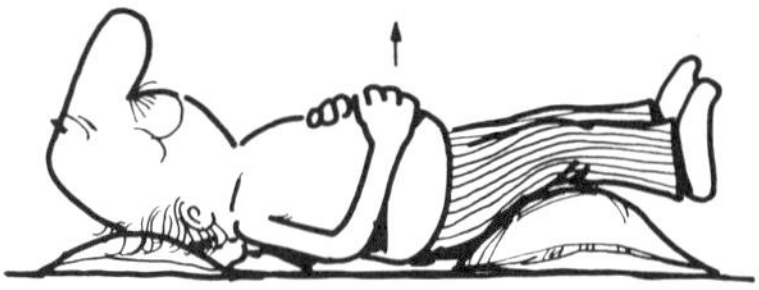

EXERCISE 2—LOWER SIDE RIB BREATHING

Assume a comfortable sitting position and good posture.

1. Place your hands on your sides at the base of your ribs.
2. Breathe out slowly through pursed lips. Your ribs should move inward (Figure C).
3. Breathe in slowly through the nose and allow ribs to expand outward against your hands (Figure D).
4. Rest.

C

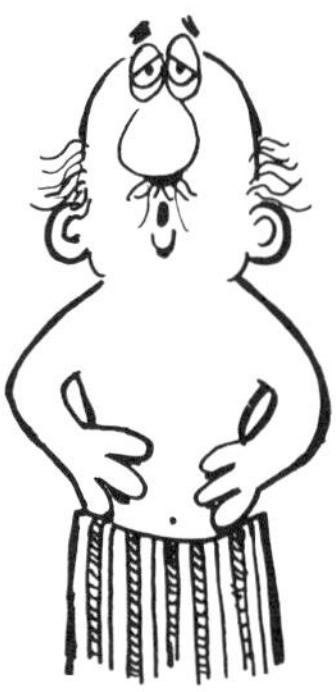

D

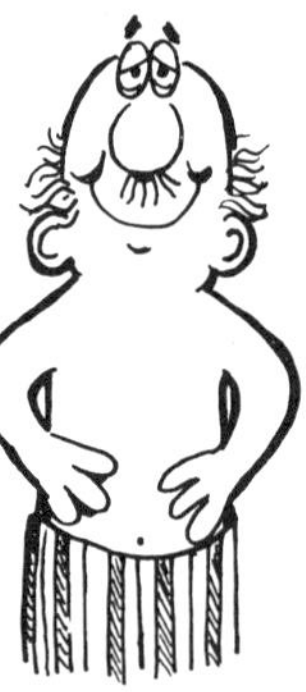

After you have mastered each of these exercises, practice combining them. It is necessary to practice often in order to strengthen and coordinate your muscles. Set aside certain times (two or three) throughout the day to practice. Be sure to rest after three or four deep breaths, or you may become lightheaded. Concentrate on making each breath slow and deep. Pursed lip breathing should always be used when practicing diaphragmatic breathing.

Diaphragmatic breathing can become your normal breathing pattern if practiced faithfully and will result in less shortness of breath. Whenever you become short of breath, diaphragmatic and pursed lip breathing should be used. They should also be used during exercise and during strenuous activities. You must master these techniques before going on to other exercises.

CONTROLLED COUGHING TECHNIQUE

Coughing is the natural way of removing foreign substances from the lungs. In COPD there is an excess production of mucus, which must be removed to maintain open airways and allow you to move air in and out of your lungs effectively. If the excess mucus is not removed, shortness of breath can worsen. Retained mucus can also contribute to the risk of infection. In addition, the mucus irritates nerve endings in the tracheobronchial tree and can cause frequent, involuntary coughing, resulting in fatigue. To conserve energy and oxygen, you must practice and master the method of controlled coughing.

STEP **1.** Take a slow deep breath, using diaphragmatic breathing. Building up a volume of air behind the mucus helps to propel it toward the mouth.

STEP **2.** Hold the deep breath for 2 seconds.

STEP **3.** Cough twice with your mouth slightly open. The first cough loosens and the second cough moves the mucus.

STEP **4.** Pause.

STEP **5.** Inhale by sniffing gently. Taking in a big breath after coughing only causes you to cough again and may drive the mucus back into the lungs.

STEP **6.** Rest.

A drink of water taken prior to coughing can be helpful. Coughing is easier when you are in a sitting position with your head slightly forward. Controlled, effective coughing should make a hollow sound.

COUGHING STEPS IN BRIEF

1. Deep breathe.
2. Hold your breath.
3. Cough twice.
4. Pause.
5. Inhale by sniffing gently.
6. Rest.

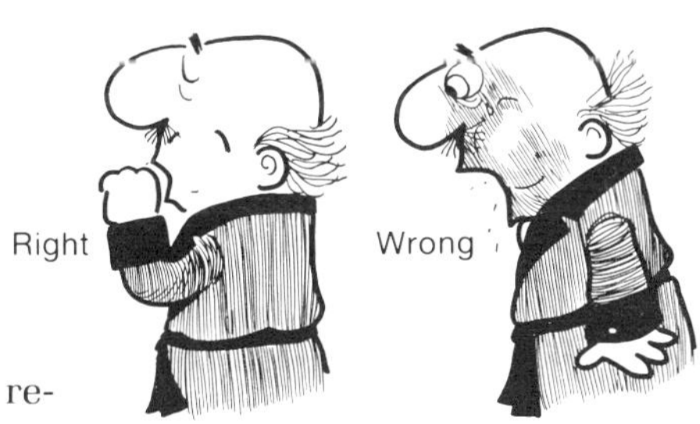

If you need to cough again, repeat the procedure step by step.

Control your cough—don't let it control you.

6 Day in, day out: your daily activities

The use of proper breathing techniques while going about your daily routine will enable you to do *more* with *less* shortness of breath. You must pace your work to your capacity and always maintain a controlled breathing pattern. If you feel like taking a couple of breaths between the work, do so—then continue as described. It is not necessary to work on every exhalation.

Rules

1. Take a deep breath by using your diaphragm before doing any work (especially something strenuous).
2. While you are exhaling (which is the most passive part of breathing), the work itself should be performed.
3. Remember to breathe out at least twice as long as you breathe in (for example, inhale 2 seconds, exhale 4 seconds).

Standing up from a chair

Take a deep breath by using your diaphragm.
While breathing out through pursed lips, rise to your feet.

Going up a flight of stairs or walking up a hill

Take a deep breath by using your diaphragm before you start to climb.
While breathing out through pursed lips, climb two or three stairs or take two or three steps.
Stop and rest while breathing in with your diaphragm again.
If you should feel short of breath at this point, then rest for a while, taking as many breaths as you need to feel comfortable again. Then continue the climbing in the same manner as just described.

Lifting loads

Take a deep breath by using your diaphragm.
While breathing out with pursed lips, lift and place load where intended.
Many people with COPD regard all arm movements, especially about the shoulders, as difficult and tiresome. The following examples show how to coordinate proper breathing with these movements.

Pushing a broom, vacuum cleaner, or lawn mower

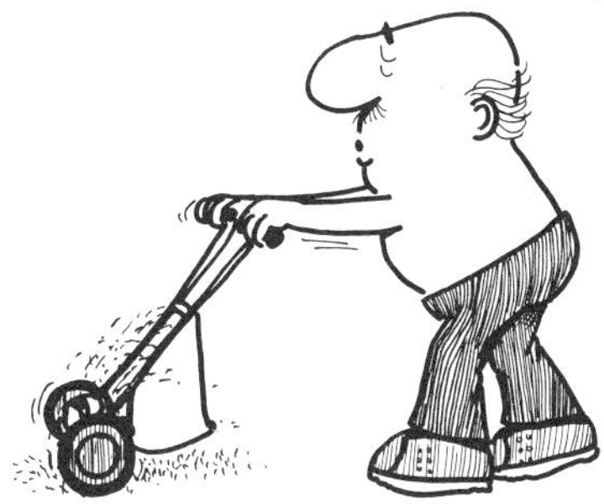

Take a deep breath by using your diaphragm before you start to push.

Push objects while breathing out with pursed lips.

Stop and rest while breathing in, using your diaphragm again. Continue your pushing in the same manner as just described.

Shaving, combing hair

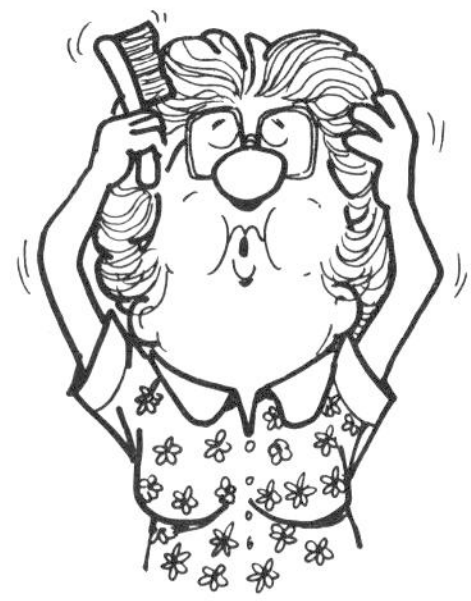

Take a deep breath by using your diaphragm.

While breathing out with pursed lips, lift your arms and shave or comb two or three strokes.

Lower your arms and rest while breathing in, using your diaphragm again.

Continue your shaving or combing in the same manner as just described.

Reaching

Take a deep breath by using your diaphragm.

While breathing out with pursed lips, lift your arms to shoulder level or above, reaching for the intended goal.

Some additional examples of when you might use this breathing technique

Household tasks

- Bedmaking
- Window washing
- Mopping
- Moving furniture
- Putting away dishes

Exercises

- Walking
- Breathing exercises
- Body improvement exercises
- Bronchial drainage
- Relaxation exercises

Garden work

- Digging
- Raking leaves
- Weeding

Hobbies

- Golfing
- Bowling

Personal hygiene

- Dressing
- Brushing teeth
- Showering

Some examples of energy-saving techniques

Economizing your energy can be important in order to complete your necessary daily chores. Often this can be accomplished by slight changes in the way you perform these tasks.

1. Plan your daily chores in advance so you won't feel rushed or have to push yourself beyond your limitations.
2. Make a decision as to which jobs are absolutely necessary to make your home comfortable and attractive.
3. Adopt a cooperative work-sharing attitude within your family. Assign tasks and responsibilities.
4. Pace all work to your own speed.
5. Distribute tedious tasks throughout the week.
6. Do the tasks requiring the most exertion when you have the most energy. For example, if mornings are difficult, take your shower and set the breakfast table the evening before.
7. Interchange the easy with the difficult activities, and take rest periods in between to prevent overfatigue.
8. When possible, sit down to work. For example, make use of a kitchen stool and a shower stool.
9. Drain dishes dry instead of towel drying.

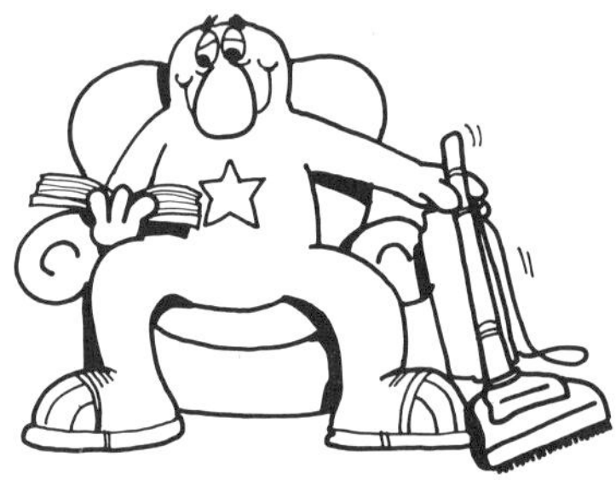

10. Prepare food for two or more meals at one cooking session. Refrigerate or freeze the additional meals for another time.
11. Unclutter your storage areas (such as cupboards, wardrobes, and tool sheds) so that you can easily find and reach what you need.
12. Avoid ironing clothes as much as possible by using drip-dry fabrics.
13. Straighten up rooms as you go along. A good rule is "never leave a room empty-handed."
14. Vacuuming may leave fine dust in the air. To prevent breathing it, tie a moist handkerchief in front of your mouth and nose while vacuuming; open windows and let the room air out for at least an hour. Use only disposable vacuum bags.
15. When making your bed, start at the head and progress down the bed toward and across the foot, tucking in and smoothing as you go. Then proceed up the second side. A bed on casters makes moving it easier; however, it is more convenient if only the head

of the bed is against the wall. Since an electric blanket is lightweight it will be easier to lift and weigh less heavily on your body at night.

Some tips for daily self-care

Your hygiene and grooming can be some of the more exerting activities you have to do in a day.

1. Caring for the hair is less work if you have a short, easy-to-maintain haircut.
2. If brushing teeth is a chore, use an electric toothbrush.
3. If you feel smothered under an overhead shower or when splashing water on your face, use a washcloth and install a hand shower in order to control the direction and force of flow.
4. If steam in the shower bothers you, try turning on the cold water first, then slowly add the hot. (Don't forget to use a stool to sit on while in the shower!)

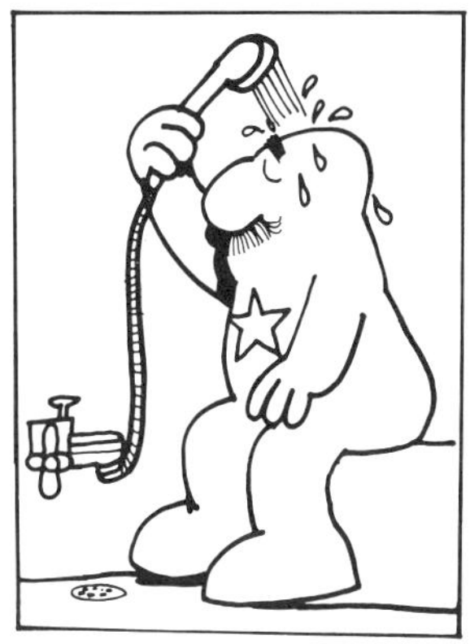

5. Putting grab bars and no-slip strips in the tub or shower will help you keep your balance.
6. Avoid all scented soaps, colognes, etc., if you find they bother your breathing.
7. In order to scrub your back, a folded towel with handles at each end and with a brush or loofah sponge attached in the middle is easy to pull diagonally back and forth across your back. This is available in most bath shops.
8. Rubbing yourself dry after a bath can be very tiring. Try wrapping yourself in a robe made of terry cloth. Its absorbent qualities will dry you "automatically."
9. Be sure to use your oxygen in the shower or bath if you have been prescribed oxygen with activity. The portable tank can be set just outside the shower or tub and extra long tubing used.
10. Do not "lock yourself up" in the bathroom. Keep windows and doors open as much as possible. Otherwise use a fan. The air does not necessarily have to be fresh for you to breathe better, as long as it circulates.

• • •

Remember, coordinate your breathing techniques with *all* of these activities:

1. Use the diaphragm and relax the accessory muscles when you breathe in.
2. Use pursed lips while you breathe out; breathe out at least twice as long as you breathe in.
3. Do strenuous work, especially work involving climbing, holding the arms up, and compressing the trunk, on exhalation only.

7 Cleaning out your tubes: bronchial drainage

Persons with chronic lung disease have secretions in their bronchial tubes, which not only make it more difficult to breathe but also may interfere with oxygen's getting into the blood. These secretions are also a perfect place for bacteria to grow and multiply and cause a major lung infection. By draining these secretions, you will be able to breathe more easily, prevent infections, and generally feel better.

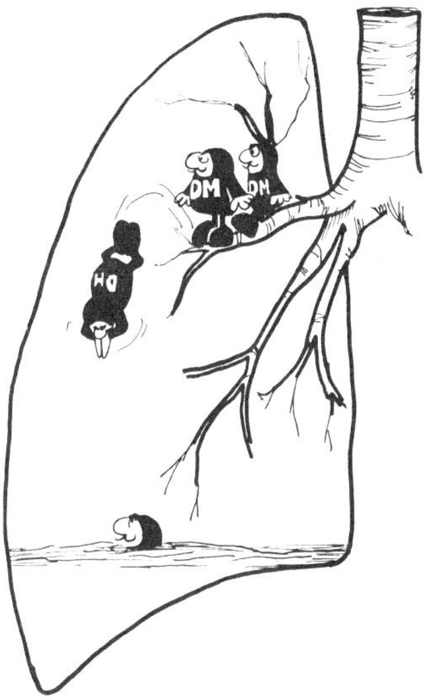

Secretions tend to pool in the bottom of your lungs because humans spend most of their time in the upright position. In order to get secretions to a point where you can cough them up more easily, you must tilt your chest so that with the assistance of gravity the bronchial tubes of the lower lung area can drain—this is bronchial drainage.

You should learn the techniques of bronchial drainage from a therapist or nurse only when ordered by your doctor. Some basic points, the steps to follow, and pictures of bronchial drainage positions will help you to remember what you have learned.

BASIC POINTS

1. It is best done first thing in the morning (1 hour before breakfast) and in the evening (at least 1 hour before bedtime).
2. Do bronchial drainage at least once or twice daily. Increase the number of treatments to three or four when your secretions change color, increase in amount, or you have a cold.
3. When you feel like doing your bronchial drainage the least, you probably need it the most.
4. It is most important to tilt the chest area 10 to 20 degrees below the

horizontal level. This can be accomplished by using one of the following suggested methods:

A slant board
An ironing board or a board 2 feet by 6 feet propped against a couch
Couch pillows placed on the floor
Firm pillows propped under your hips in bed
A positional lounge chair

There is no excuse for skipping your bronchial drainage!

STEPS TO FOLLOW FOR EFFECTIVE BRONCHIAL DRAINAGE

STEP **1.** *Conditioning of airways and secretions*

Take prescribed medications to dilate your airways before you begin bronchial drainage. Inhaled bronchodilator medicine should be taken 10 minutes before doing bronchial drainage. Oral bronchodilator medicine should ideally be taken at least 30 minutes beforehand.

Drink *at least* 1½ quarts of liquid daily. Adequate fluid intake is mandatory to keep mucus thin. Breathe in moist air (from IPPB machines, nebulizers, vaporizers, a warm shower, or boiling water placed in a bowl). These techniques also help to make mucus thin.

STEP **2.** *Good inflation of the lungs*

Breathing exercises are *extremely* important. Diaphragmatic and pursed lip breathing should be done throughout the bronchial drainage period. They help widen your airways so secretions can be drained.

STEP **3.** *Use of gravity, percussion, and vibration*

The use of gravity is the most important aspect of draining secretions. The positions on the next page show gravity drainage positions. Stay in each of the positions (1 through 4) for 5 to 15 minutes.

Percussion and vibration are additional methods of loosening secretions. Percussion may be prescribed for at least 1 minute in each position. Percussion, or clapping with a cupped hand on the chest wall, helps to move secretions into larger airways. Percussion should be done only on the rib cage and not over the spinal column, breastbone, or soft tissues.

Vibration is the other means of moving secretions. Your rib cage may be vibrated by another person or a mechanical device. Vibration should follow percussion and is done for an additional minute only when you are exhaling.

Your skin should be covered with clothing or a towel during

Bronchial drainage positions
Daily routine

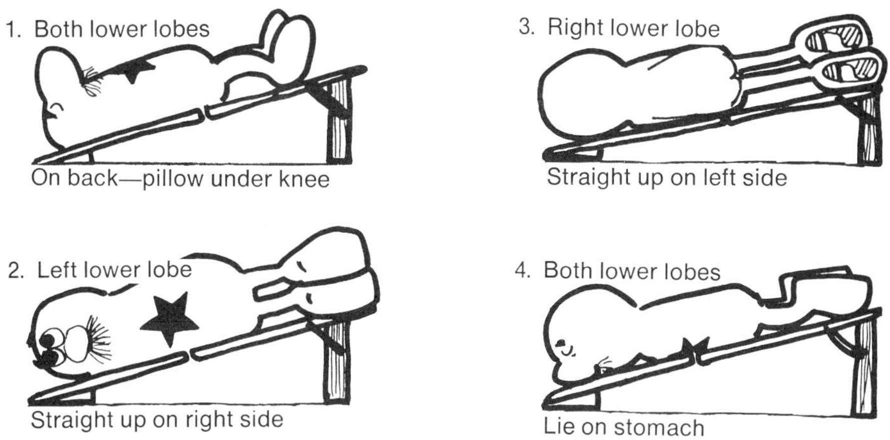

percussion and vibration. Your doctor or therapist should instruct you in these procedures.

If additional positions are needed, your doctor, therapist, or nurse will prescribe them.

STEP **4.** *Controlled coughing*

Remember to cough after each position. Use the controlled coughing technique. Rest after coughing.

PRECAUTIONS

If you have high blood pressure or a heart problem, be sure to check with your doctor before doing bronchial drainage. If you are on steroids or have osteoporosis (weak bones), check with your doctor before doing percussion or vibration on your chest.

1. Condition airways and secretions.
2. Inflate lungs.
3. Use gravity drainage.
4. Cough after each position.

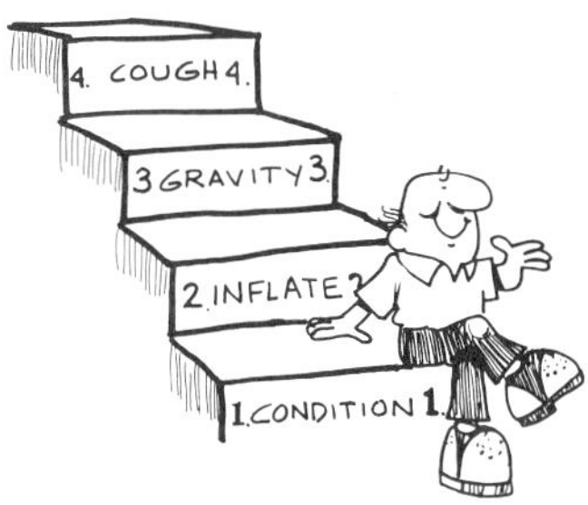

8 The joy of exercise

FIRST THINGS FIRST

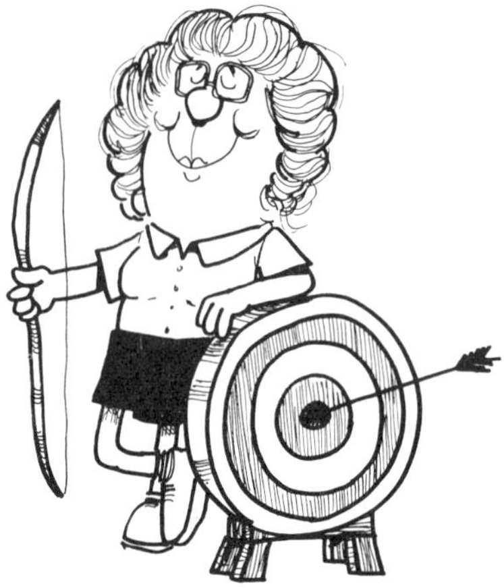

Good physical condition is an objective that everyone should seek; the patient with COPD is no exception. Many COPD patients, having had their lung problems for several years, may have avoided much physical activity because of the limitations imposed by the shortness of breath. In addition, friends, family, or physicians may have encouraged them not to exert themselves, assuming that to do so might cause "harmful effects." After years of study we now know this isn't true. *Inactivity* is an *enemy* working *against* you! Sitting or lying around deconditions the body and makes all of your muscles less strong, less efficient. This, in turn, makes doing even the simplest daily activities more difficult, energy-wise and breathing-wise. This deconditioning effect can be reversed by a regular exercise program. The three major systems involved in exercise are the skeletal muscles, specialized heart muscles, and respiratory muscles. By progressive exercise of any kind, the fibers of the muscles involved become more efficient; that is, they need less and less oxygen for the same amount of work. Thus, you may have more "energy" to accomplish the tasks you perform each day.

The reconditioning of muscles should be undertaken with great care, since suddenly starting to exercise may be useless at best and hazardous at worst. The proper way to approach improving your physical condition depends on two fundamentals:

1. The goals you seek
2. Your overall health at the time you start a physical conditioning program

Someone whose goal is to win the Olympic mile run, and who is 18 years old with no health limitations, can enter a program that consists of running more and more miles each week at a faster and faster pace. This program, like all conditioning programs, will be progressive; that is, it will increase in distance and speed until the maximum tolerable level is reached.

Weightlifters, on the other hand, would start a progressive program of muscle-building that involves techniques quite unlike those used by a runner. Gymnasts and ballet dancers, again, would follow different routines. They too need conditioning. But for *their* goals, different muscles are involved, and they seek body flexibility as well as endurance and strength. A physical conditioning program designed for a weightlifter might ruin the career of a gymnast or ballet dancer.

Furthermore, a program developed for a young athlete can be hazardous for an individual who has a known (or unknown) health problem. A 50-year-old man who has decided to enter the "Senior Olympics" should devise his physical conditioning program with great caution and under close medical guidance. Otherwise, a heart attack (rather than a new world record) can be his reward. Similar cautions apply to the Sunday tennis player who in 90-degree temperatures is carried away by the contest, failing to recognize that he or she has not exercised regularly during prior weeks (or months).

So, regardless of the individual involved, the goals of the program and consideration of overall health status should precede the starting of a physical conditioning program.

Like the different types of athletes, patients with COPD should set specific goals involving the physical activities that they would like to achieve. These goals should be realistic and, preferably, written down.

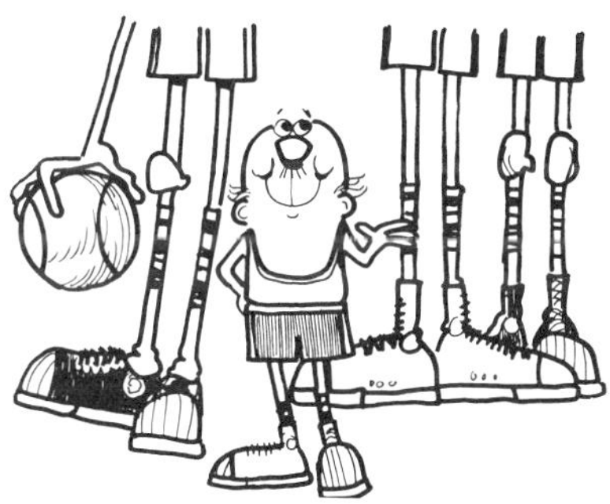

In goal-setting, the athlete is limited by his natural abilities, body build, and motivation. A 4-foot, 10-inch athlete should not aim at being a star professional basketball center. The patient with COPD is also subject to these limitations in goal-setting, plus an additional one: the status of his lung function. Careful evaluation of the type and extent of lung function abnormalities present is essential before establishing a physical conditioning program. Such evaluation is required for two reasons:

1. Certain specific physical conditioning techniques can be undertaken in the COPD patient to improve lung function itself.
2. The status of lung function must be known to establish safe limits of exercise.

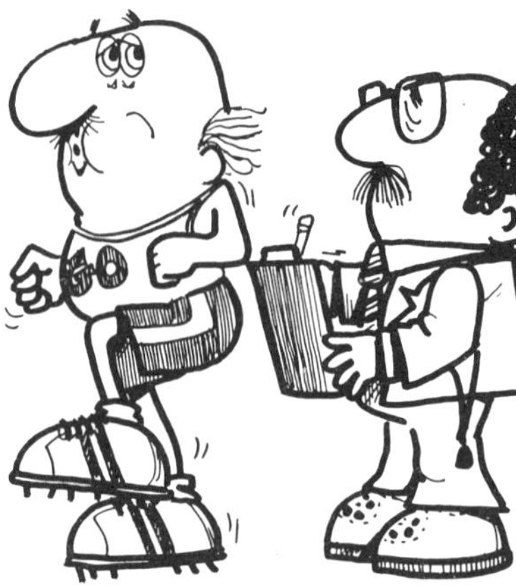

PLAY IT SAFE

Your doctor will choose the methods of evaluating your "exercise tolerance" and work with you to choose the type of exercise that is most useful and best fits in with your life-style.

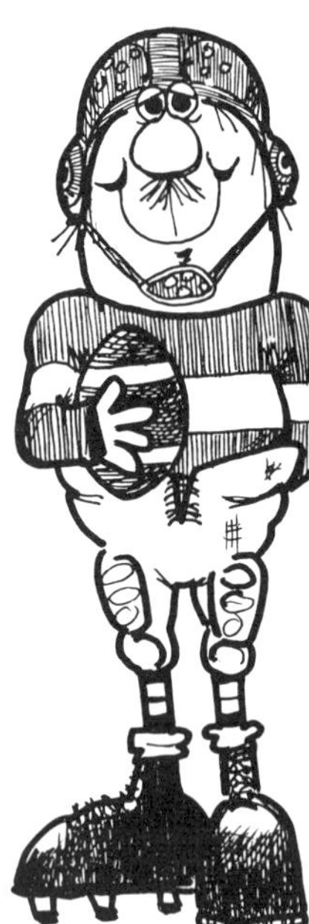

Each part of your physical conditioning program should be checked for safety *before* you attempt it. This is not a responsibility you should assume. For example, walking too far too quickly may put excessive strain on your lungs or heart. Or certain activities may cause your blood oxygen level to fall to undesirable levels. So do not attempt to construct your own program. Your doctor will do that with you. Your doctor wants to get you in optimal condition—but within the limits he knows to be safe. These limits can be established only by testing, then by tailoring your program to your specific lung, heart, and other limitations. There are no simple guidelines that you yourself can establish. For instance, becoming short of breath during a given exercise does *not* mean that you are overdoing and have to stop. If it did, most athletes would stop in the middle of a race, a tennis match, or a football game. Even fatigue or aching muscles do not necessarily mean you are overdoing. It may be necessary to experience such discomforts to improve your condition. So let your physician set the limits, based on his detailed knowledge of your condition.

TYPES OF EXERCISE

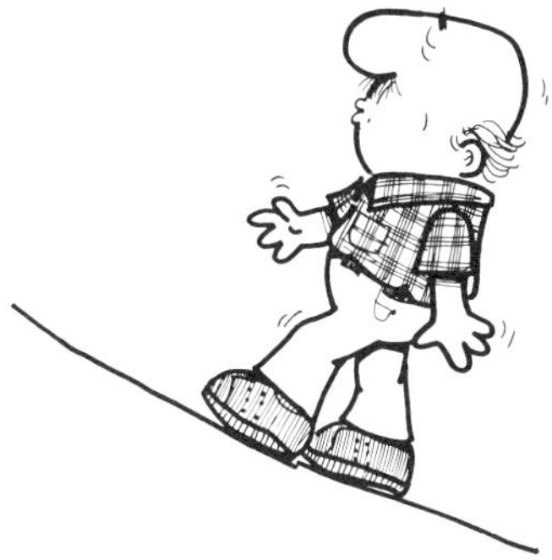

The kind of exercise that will benefit you most depends on what you want to do. What does that mean? It means that exercise training is rather specific: weight-lifting, swimming, bicycling, running, dancing, jumping, calisthenics, etc., all "train" different muscles. Most patients with COPD want to increase their ability to walk in terms of both speed and distance. In fact, walking is one of the best forms of exercise because: (1) it uses many body muscles, including the heart and diaphragm; (2) it requires no special equipment or skill; and (3) it can be measured easily (speed, distance). Therefore, walking is the usual starting point for most COPD patients. From this starting point you may want to branch out to other types of exercise.

YOUR JOB

Whatever the exercise program designed for you, *you* will be responsible for mastering it. You will find that you may have to push yourself some to establish a regular routine. Being short of breath creates a big temptation to remain inactive, especially on the days when the shortness of breath may seem worse. Keep a careful record of your exercise sessions—for example, how long you walked, how fast you walked, your pulse rate before and after, and how you tolerated the exercise. Then, you and your doctor can monitor your progress and adjust your exercise routine as necessary.

Your doctor and other health professionals will guide you. But then it is *your job* to pick up the ball and carry through by following the program regularly.

9 Letting go: relaxation techniques

WHY TALK ABOUT RELAXATION?

When you are physically and emotionally relaxed, excessive oxygen consumption caused by tension of overworked muscles is avoided. Relaxation also decreases other undesirable manifestations of stress such as mental irritability and anxiety that might induce bronchospasm, increased shortness of breath, and fatigue. By using some of the suggested relaxation methods outlined below, you can relieve the tension that increases your respiratory difficulties. Complete muscular relaxation is also important to gain maximum benefits from all other exercises.

The key to relaxation is, above all, breathing control. When you can master diaphragmatic breathing, relaxation of the accessory muscles, and prolonged exhalation with pursed lips at times of stress, you have achieved a major victory in the battle against panic. At such times, also remember positioning, which can be either standing or sitting, but always leaning forward with your arms supported.

To practice this first progressive relaxation technique, lie down on a comfortable surface and place a pillow under your head and knees. Quiet, peaceful surroundings are helpful. The principle that applies here is that maximum relaxation follows maximum contraction.

HEAD AND NECK

Pull chin down toward chest as tightly as possible and push back of head into pillow, then let go.

Turn head from side to side in a relaxed manner. Let it stop when it comes to a comfortable position.

SHOULDERS

Shrug shoulders and tighten the shoulder muscles as much as possible, then let go.

ARMS

Do one hand and one arm at a time.

Bend elbow and make a fist out of your hand. Tighten as much as possible, then let go. Straighten arm and fingers. Tighten as much as possible, then let go.

LEGS

Do one leg at a time.

Straighten leg and point toe; tighten as much as possible, then let go. Pull toes toward your nose and push heel and back of leg into bed. Tighten as much as possible, then let go.

BACK

Arch your back up like a cat. Do not lift your hips while arching. Tighten as much as possible, then let go.

FACE

Tighten (scrinch) all of your face muscles. Hold, then let go.

EYES

Try to focus your eyes on something. Watch it and slowly let your eyelids grow heavy. Open your eyes and let them close gradually until they feel comfortable closed.

Sweet dreams!

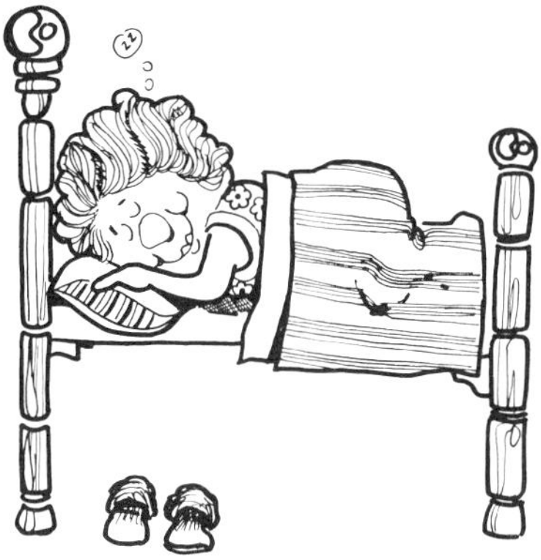

OTHER RELAXATION TECHNIQUES

Another way to control your tension is to create, in your mind, a mental picture of something that gives you a good and comfortable feeling. This may be a scene, real or imagined; a landscape with rolling hills, green grass, and trees with their leaves gently moving in the wind; or the beach, a poolside, or your mother's kitchen. Try to make your mental picture detailed. Each time you find yourself physically in a difficult situation that you cannot immediately leave (for example, a crowded elevator), use the visual image you have created as a mental escape. This will help keep your anxiety and shortness of breath under control until you can physically remove yourself from that situation.

"Mind-over-matter" relaxation techniques are another way to help increase your mind's awareness and control over your body. There are many different ways to do this type of "self-hypnosis." You can simply concentrate on a certain part of your body; for instance, concentrate on your right hand, and envision that it is becoming very limp, soft, heavy, or light. Any of these sensations will induce relaxation. Sometimes during a stressful or anxiety-provoking event, blood will rush to the center of the body, leaving the limbs cool and moist. Thinking of your hands and feet as "getting warm" is very effective, since relaxation will occur when the temperature increases. Try it first with one hand and, when you have

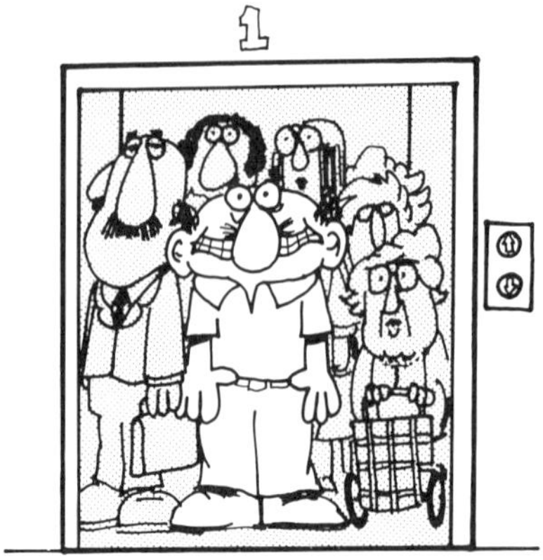

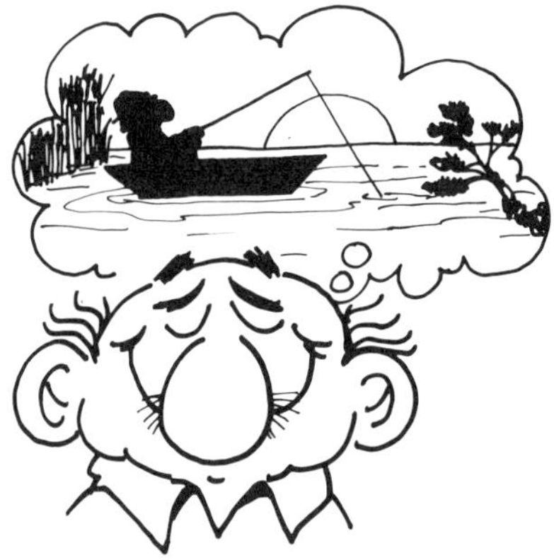

succeeded in warming it, proceed up the arm, then to the shoulder, then to the other hand, and so on until you have finally "told" your whole body to relax and it has obeyed you.

Another useful relaxation technique is one most frequently used in different types of meditation. Concentrate on one word and repeat it over and over to yourself (such as the word "free"). Repeat the word each time you breathe out. Do not let yourself get distracted by intruding thoughts; ignore them and return to repeating your word. Don't be concerned about how deep a relaxation level you are reaching. When trying these different modes of relaxation exercises, become passive and allow relaxaton to come about at its own pace.

Sleep eradicates the effects of daily fatigue. Many people with COPD, however, have trouble sleeping, sometimes because of their medications. The events of modern life, in addition, frequently overload human faculties, causing exhaustion that may not be corrected by sleep. Meditation is thought to produce an extraordinarily deep rest and a stress release much more complete than sleep. It is particularly suited for gradual removal of long-accumulated stress. This might be one relaxation method you would want to investigate further. Meditation can be used in conjunction with the progressive relaxation technique first mentioned. You start by relaxing your muscles, then you meditate.

Other modes of relaxation can include learning to give yourself a massage or having your spouse give you one, especially on the neck and shoulder muscles. The vibrator you use for bronchial drainage can be very useful for this purpose also (see Chapter 7). Biofeedback is another way to learn to relax and explore your own ability to control tension and shortness of breath. You might have already found your own way to relax, be it soft music, yoga, or a bubble bath. There are many simple techniques worth trying. If they work for you, use them!

10 Making your body work better

BODY IMPROVEMENT EXERCISES

The techniques described here will not help the lungs themselves but will improve your entire physical condition. These body improvement exercises will increase the efficiency of your muscles so that they require less fuel (oxygen) during exertion.

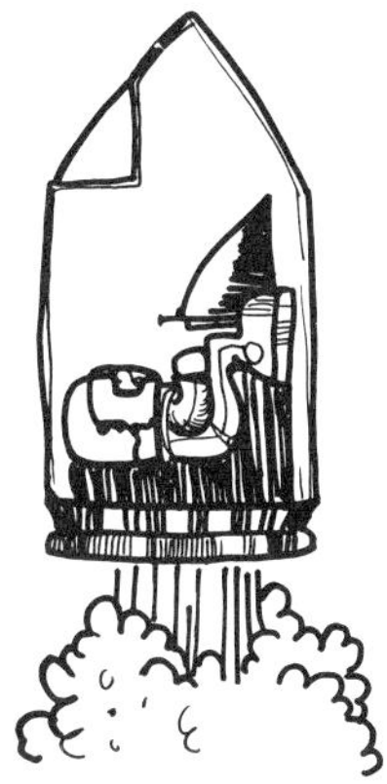

Before starting on these exercises, you want to be sure that your lungs are as "clean" as possible. So if you have excess mucus, you should clear your lungs of mucus by the techniques already described before beginning these exercises. If you are tense, total body relaxation techniques should be followed before exercise. And if pursed lip breathing or diaphragmatic breathing has been prescribed for you, you should use these methods *during* exercise.

In other words, you should have "all systems go" before "blasting off" into body improvement exercises. This is like the athlete who warms up before his event. Once you are warmed up, you can get started!

Each exercise may be done daily two to five times *after* first checking with your physician or therapist regarding your specific physical limitations (see Chapter 8).

Exercises to strengthen abdominal muscles

Some patients with COPD must work to get air out as well as in. Strong abdominal muscles can help push air out by compressing the rib cage and pulling the lower ribs downward. Through active exercise the abdominal muscles can regain their elasticity and their capacity to relax. This aids diaphragmatic breathing and also effective coughing.

CONTRACTION OF ABDOMINAL MUSCLES
WITH PELVIC TILT

1. Lie on your back with knees bent and feet flat on the floor. Place a pillow under your head (basic starting position, Figure A).
2. While exhaling, contract the abdominal muscles and roll your hips

under so that the back is flat against the floor (Figure B).
3. Relax your muscles and rest.
4. Repeat.

A

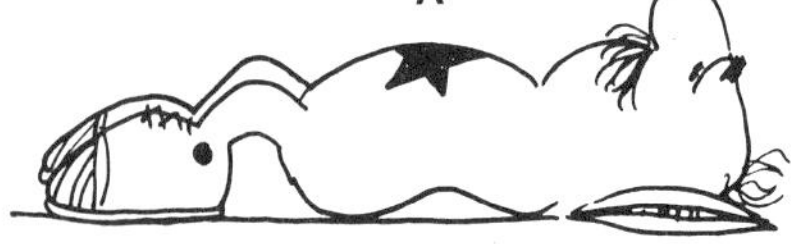

Note: If you are unable to contract your abdominal muscles as described, start your exercise program with any of the following exercises until you gain awareness of the state of your abdominal muscles and how to use them.

B

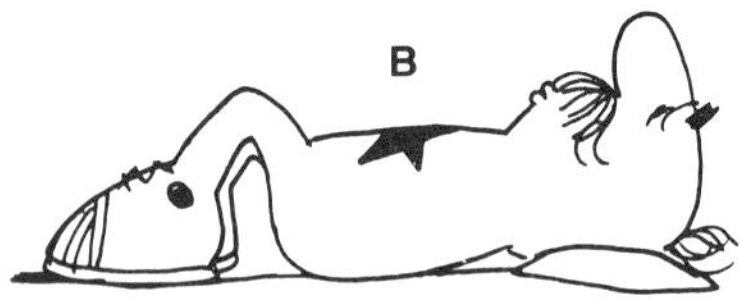

HEAD AND SHOULDER RAISING

1. Assume basic starting position and place your hands behind your head.
2. With your chin tucked in and while exhaling, raise your head and shoulders as far as you can.
3. Return to starting position and rest.
4. Repeat once.

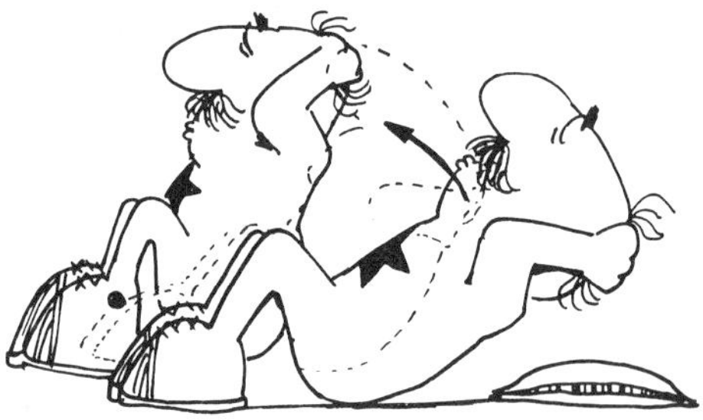

This exercise should be done smoothly to be most beneficial. As you raise your shoulders, you should contract your stomach muscles and press the small of your back against the floor. As you gain strength by doing this exercise, you may be able to curl all the way up to a sitting position. This exercise is always done on exhalation.

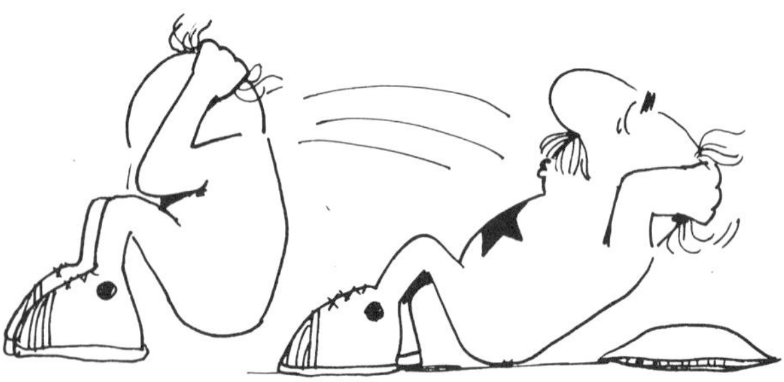

KNEE BENDING

1. Assume basic starting position shown in Figure A.
2. While exhaling, bring the left knee toward your left shoulder and press the small of the back against the floor (Figure B).
3. Return to starting position and relax.
4. Repeat on right side.

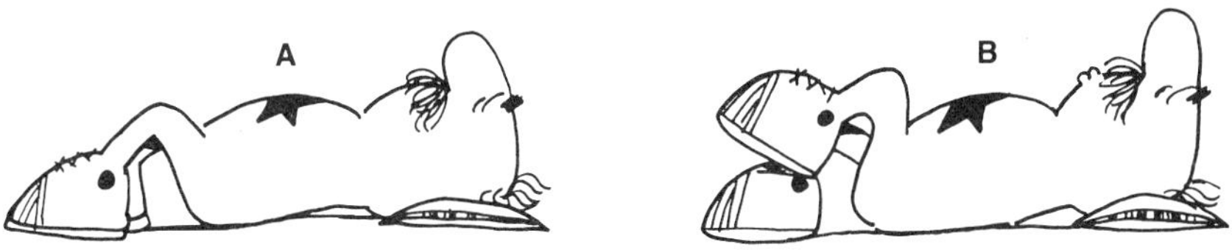

KNEE BEND WITH SHOULDER RAISE

1. Assume basic starting position with hands behind head.
2. While exhaling, raise head and shoulders as you bend your left knee toward your right shoulder.
3. Return to starting position and relax.

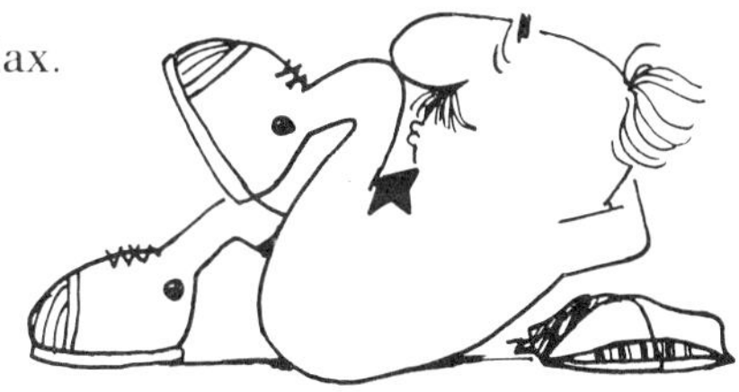

Exercises to strengthen the arms

Since arm movements can be very strenuous for patients with COPD, it is important to maintain the muscle strength with simple arm exercises. Start these by holding 1-pound dumbbells or No. 2 food cans in your hands. As you become stronger, you can increase the weight. Work both arms simultaneously, maintaining the muscle tension as you do each exercise; do not suddenly relax or drop the arms. All arm movements are done on exhalation only. (Follow the figures for each exercise.)

STRAIGHT ARM RAISES BACKWARD AND FORWARD (figure on top of p. 56)

1. Lie on your back with knees bent, feet flat on floor, arms at sides, and weights in hands.
2. Holding arms straight, lift them up and back as far as possible above your head.
3. Reverse the movement by bringing the straight arms forward and down again by your sides.
4. Repeat slowly five times, then rest.

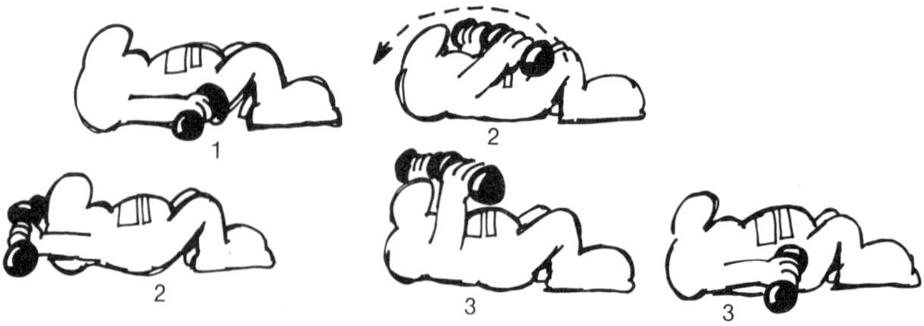

ELBOW BENDS WITH ARMS UP

1. Assume same starting position as in exercise above.
2. Bend the elbows.

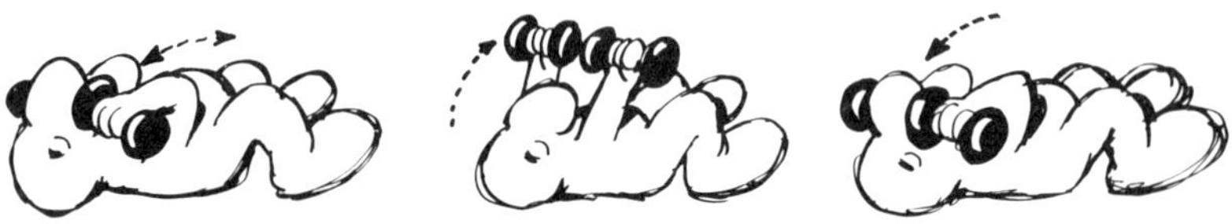

3. Straighten arms up in the air.
4. Repeat five times, then rest.

STRAIGHT ARM RAISES INWARD AND OUTWARD

1. Lie with your arms at a 90-degree angle from your body (straight out from the sides).
2. Lift both arms straight up so your hands meet above your face.
3. Keeping arms straight, return to original position.
4. Repeat five times, then rest.

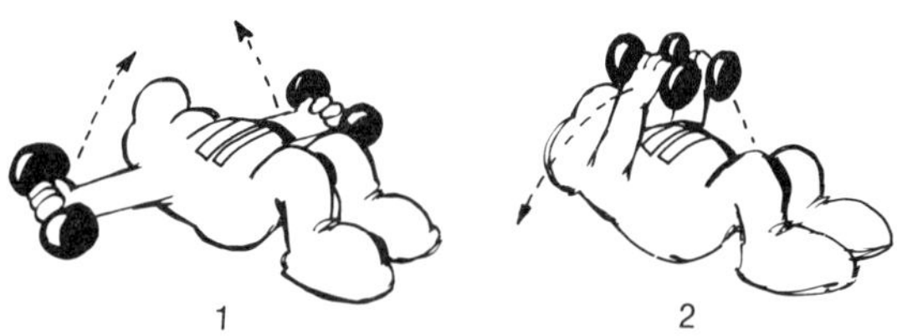

Exercises to increase mobility of the rib cage

Some patients with COPDs develop stiff rib cages, especially the lower ribs. If this is a problem, the following group of exercises will help to increase the mobility of the rib cage. This enables the lower lung areas to expand more fully.

FORWARD BENDING

1. Sit in a straight-back chair, feet flat on the floor and apart, shoulders relaxed, arms comfortable at the sides (Figure A).
2. While exhaling, drop head to your chest and slowly roll your body forward, toward your knees (Figure B). Do not jackknife at the waist (Figure C).
3. Return to the upright position slowly by pushing first the lower, then middle, then upper back against the chair.
4. Relax, inhale, then repeat.

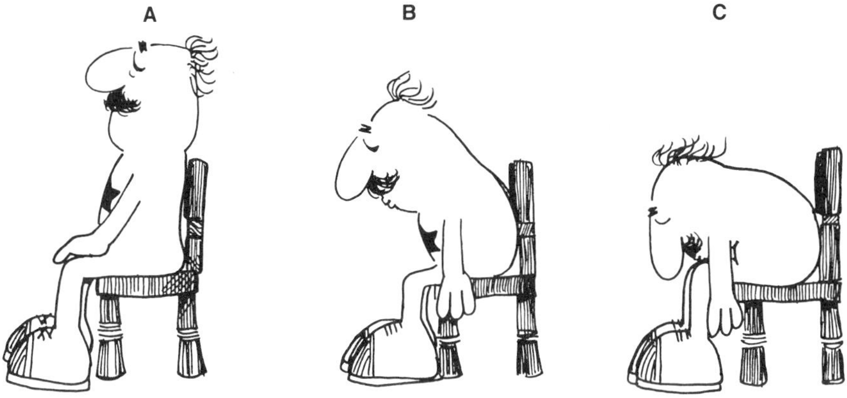

TRUNK TURNING WITH SHOULDER LOOSENING

1. Assume the same position as in the previous exercise (Figure A).
2. Turn trunk to the left while swinging outstretched arms over left shoulder, as if reaching back (Figure B). Your head should follow the movement of your hands.

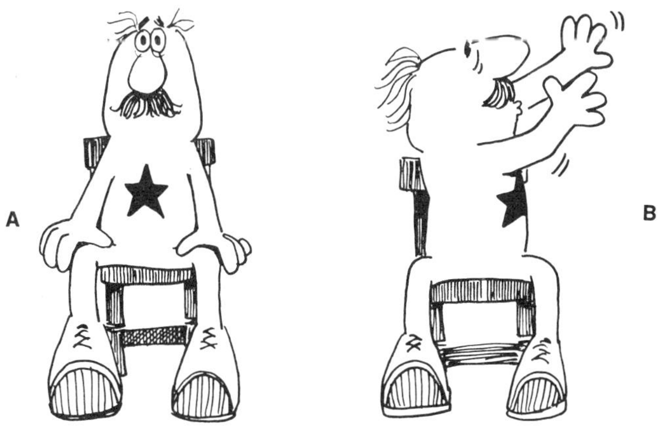

3. Return to starting position and rest.
4. Repeat on other side.

CHEST MUSCLE LOOSENING WITH BROOM

1. Sit straight, feet flat and apart, and place a broomstick comfortably on your shoulders with your arms draped over it (as shown). Do not press the broomstick hard against the spine.
2. Using a rowing motion, rotate the broom (Figure A).
3. Rest.
4. Twist the broom from side to side using only the shoulders and arms and upper trunk (Figure B).
5. Rest.
6. Repeat.

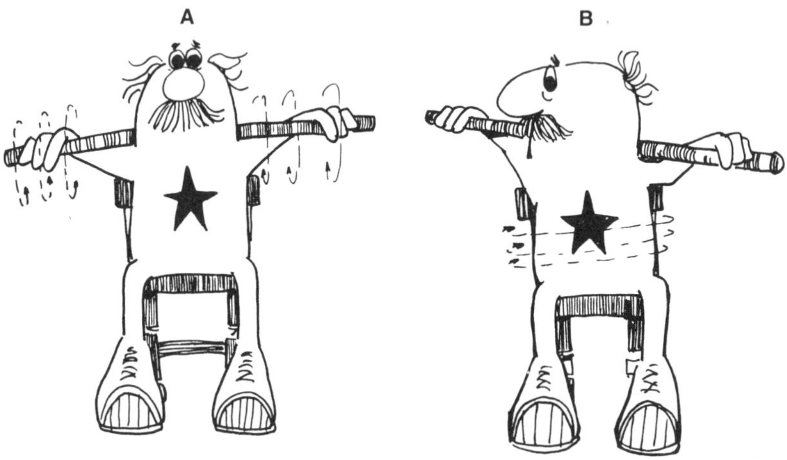

SIDE BENDING (figure on top of p. 59)

1. Sit up straight with feet apart. Place left hand on lower left rib cage and place right hand on top.
2. While exhaling slowly, bend head and shoulders to the left while pressing hands against left side (Figure A).
3. Then while inhaling, and in a continuous motion, bend the head and shoulders slightly to the right while expanding the left lower ribs as much as possible (Figure B).
4. Return to starting position and rest.
5. Repeat on other side.

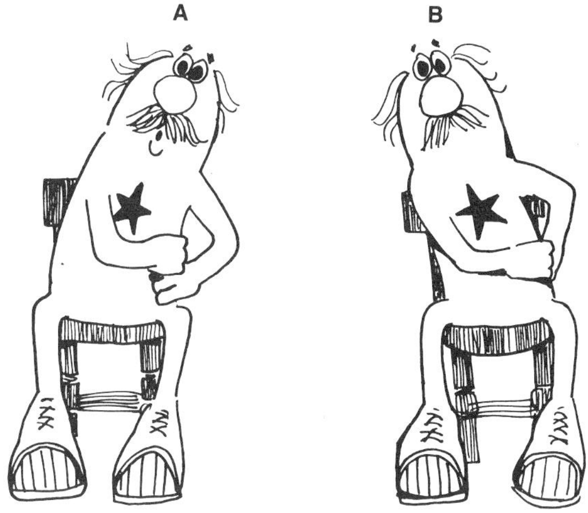

Exercises to relax shoulder and neck muscles

The shoulder and neck muscles are considered accessory respiratory muscles and are not normally involved in the work of quiet breathing. In some COPDs there is a tendency to breathe shallowly using upper chest muscles because of the decreased mobility of the rib cage and the flattening of the diaphragm. To breathe properly, you must relax your shoulder and neck muscles. The following exercises can be done anytime during the day when you feel tense in the shoulder and neck area. They should also be done between the other exercises in your program.

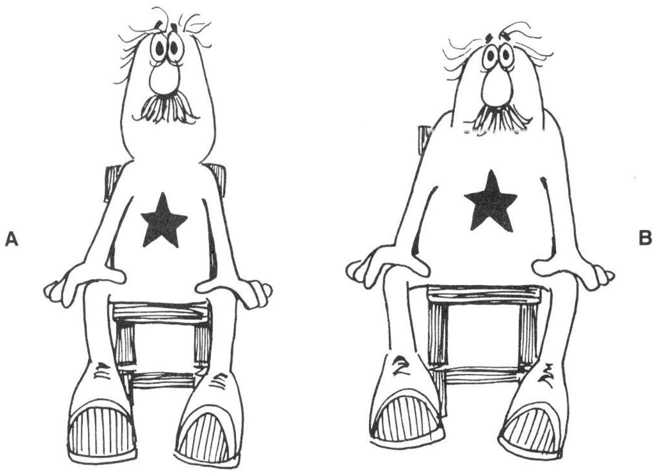

Shoulder shrugging (see p. 60)

SHOULDER SHRUGGING (figure on bottom of p. 59)

1. Stand or sit with feet slightly apart and arms relaxed.
2. Shrug shoulders and tighten the muscles as much as possible.
3. Relax and rest.
4. Repeat.

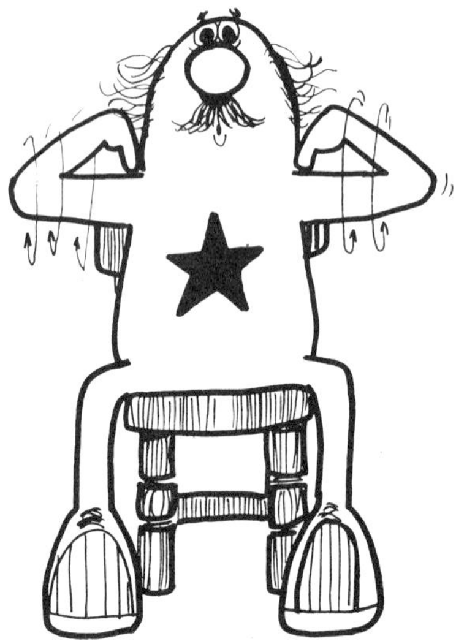

ELBOW CIRCLING

1. Sit or stand with hands on shoulders.
2. Circle the elbows forward, up, back, and downward. Do four to eight circles.
3. Relax muscles.

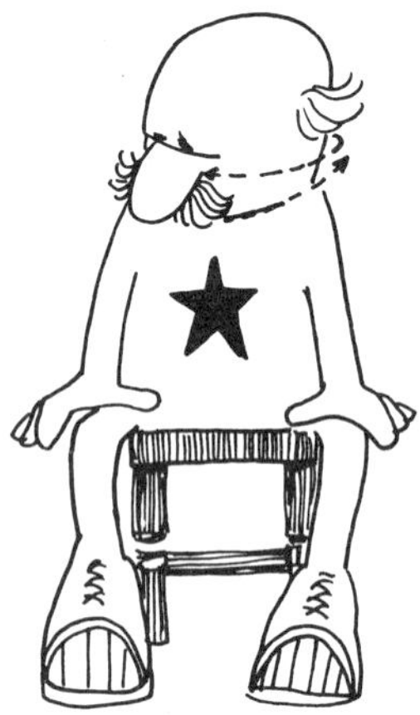

HEAD CIRCLING

1. Roll head loosely from side to side in a forward semicircle.

CIRCLING OF SHOULDERS WITH HANGING ARMS

1. Sit or stand with arms relaxed.
2. Circle left shoulder up and back.
3. Repeat on right side.
4. Finally circle both shoulders together.

A B

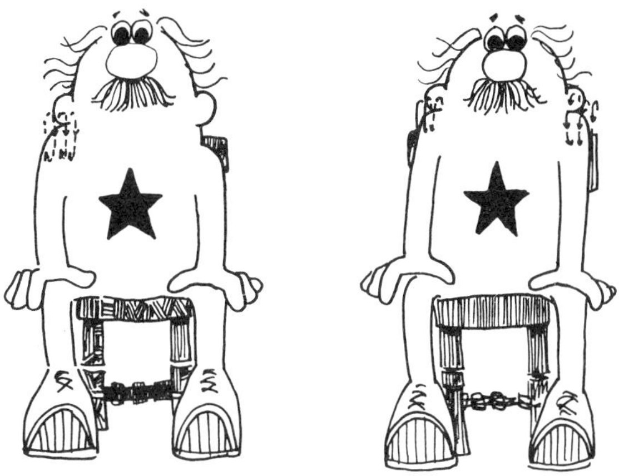

ARM SWINGING

1. Stand in straight position.
2. Swing arms forward and backward briskly (Figure A).
3. Rest.
4. Stand, bending forward slightly.
5. Swing arms loosely from side to side with hands heavy and limp (Figure B).

A B

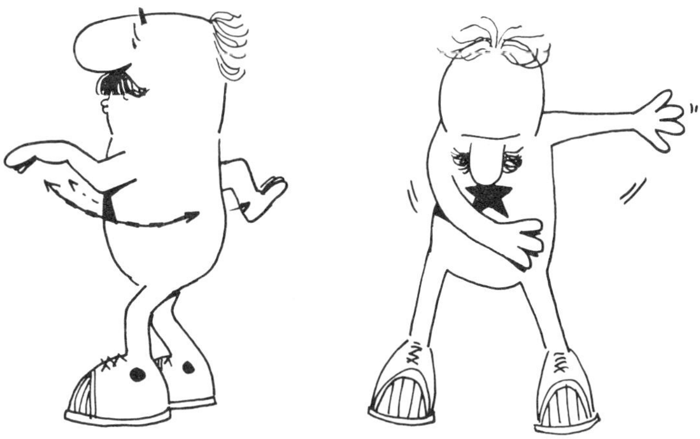

BODY MECHANICS

The joints and bones in your body are parts of a machine that will wear out if they are strained too much or incorrectly. Also, advancing age and long-term use of steroids may make bones brittle. Proper body mechanics are essential to make the whole of your body function effectively.

It is important that your motions be smooth and steady, never jerky or sudden. Do not lift, push, or pull when your back is twisted or bent. Use your *feet* to turn around, and lift by bending and straightening your knees. When you lift an object, it should be held as close to your body as possible.

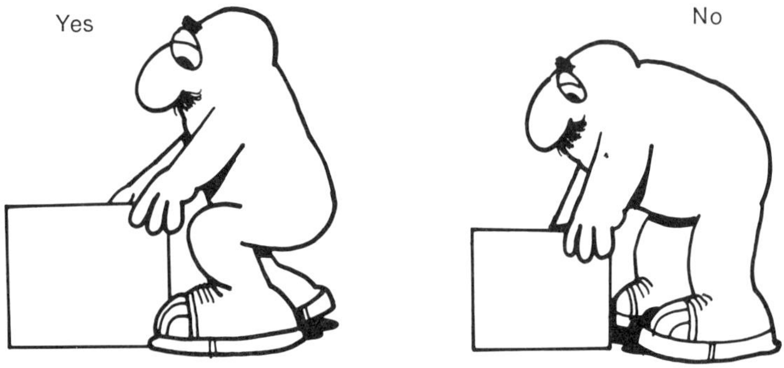

Pushing

Avoid carrying heavy items in your arms; instead, utilize a rolling cart of some kind for them (for example, groceries, laundry, equipment).

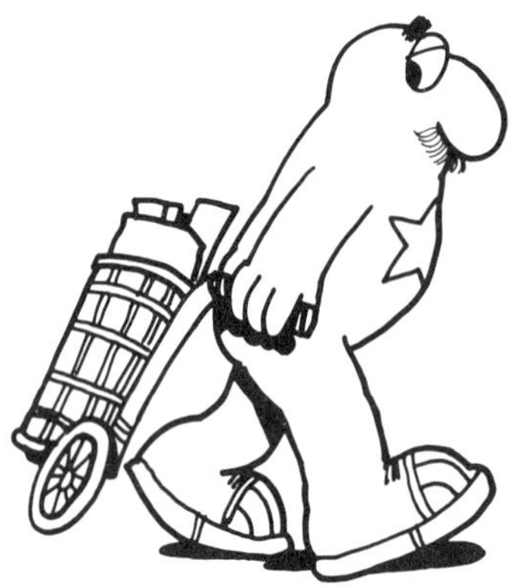

Working surfaces should be of the proper height in order to avoid excessive bending of your back or having to lift your arms too high. Proper working area height is generally a couple of inches below your elbows, for both the standing and sitting positions.

Never sit in a chair that's too low; have your back, feet, and arms well supported. You will generally feel more comfortable sitting erect or even leaning slightly forward.

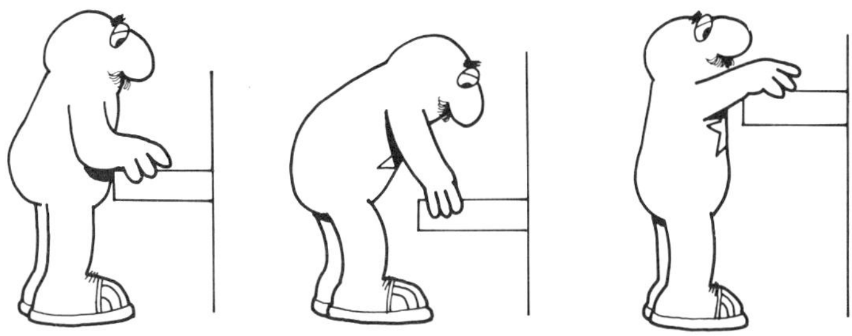

Yes No No

REDEVELOPMENT OF GOOD POSTURE

Maintaining a well-balanced carriage is as essential to habitual good breathing as using your diaphragm and abdominal muscles and relaxing the shoulders, neck, and upper chest. The following basic points should be considered and practiced.

1. Stand with at least half the body weight carried forward over the forepart of the feet so that the toes are well pressed onto the ground.
2. Practice rocking forward until the heels have to come off the ground and backward until the toes do, then settle between these two extremes. The weight should be at least evenly divided between the front of the foot and the heel. In most cases it is necessary to accentuate the forward-shifting of the weight.
3. Stand sideways in front of a long mirror and note:
   a. Is your head poking forward? Correct this by stretching upward and tucking your chin in while pressing your head backward.
   b. Is your seat sticking out? Tuck in the seat muscles and relax your shoulders and upper chest.
   c. Do your shoulders hunch forward? Bring your shoulder blades down and back.

4. When sitting in a chair, sit well back in the seat, support your legs on the floor (never dangle). Support your arms on armrests or place them on your lap.

Practice posture work against a wall for about 5 minutes at a time. Assume the following position.

1. Place feet a few inches apart a few inches away from the wall.
2. Hold head high.
3. Tuck chin in.
4. Relax shoulders.
5. Tuck hips under.
6. Slightly flex knees.

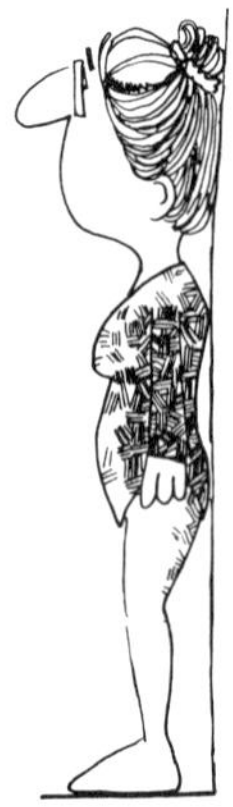

When you feel you can hold the position properly, try standing away from the wall in the proper postural position, and then attempt to walk in this position. You will notice that the trunk stays quite rigid but the legs, both hips and knees, bend more when walking in this way. Check to see if you have retained the proper position by backing up to the wall frequently during your walking practice. Do not stiffen up when trying to maintain a proper posture. Only by being relaxed can you benefit from this exercise.

11 You are what you eat

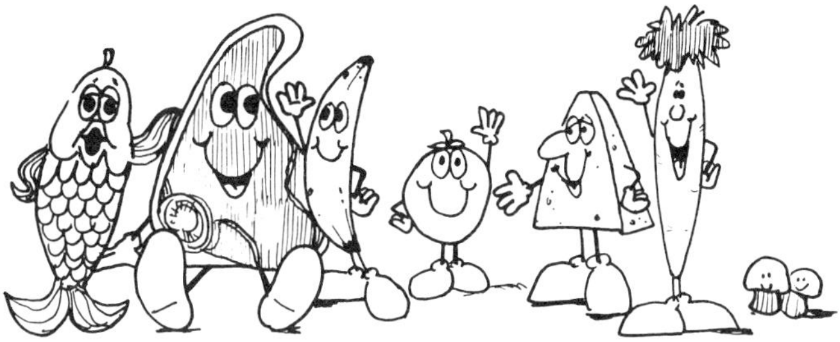

Eating good food is one of the great pleasures in life. What you eat affects the way you feel, your ability to fight infections and diseases, your emotional health, and, ultimately, the length of your life.

With decreased physical activity, you need fewer calories to burn for energy; yet you still need protein, vitamins, and minerals. You can manage this balancing act by eliminating the foods that provide mainly calories but few nutrients, such as sweets, fast foods, and packaged "goodies." Give some thought to your choices and select those foods that give you more of the nutrients you need.

THE SIX ESSENTIAL NUTRIENTS

The food you eat supplies the six nutrients necessary for life.

1. *Water* accounts for more than two thirds of your total weight. It is present in every body cell. It helps you digest food and eliminate waste. It is especially important for COPD patients to drink plenty of fluids.

2. *Protein* provides the eight essential amino acids your body needs for repairing its tissues. Milk and milk products, eggs, meat, poultry, and fish are complete proteins that contain all eight of the essential amino acids—the building materials the body cannot make for itself. Whole-grain breads and cereals, nuts, legumes, and dried beans provide useful but less complete proteins. When combined with some protein from an animal source, these "incomplete" proteins become complete with all the essential amino acids and are fully utilized by the body.

3. *Carbohydrates* are a major source of energy. They provide about 50% of the calories in the American diet. They are the cheapest and most easily digested form of energy. All tissues require glucose (a *simple* carbohydrate) as their source of energy. The *complex* carbohydrates pro-

vided by fruits, grains, potatoes, cereals, and pastas provide good quality carbohydrate as well as other nutrients. The indigestible fiber in these complex carbohydrates also provides the necessary bulk for good elimination. Simple sugars, such as table sugar, honey, and syrup, provide mainly calories.

4. *Fats* are primarily a source of energy. They provide the essential fatty acids and act as carriers for the fat-soluble vitamins (A, D, E, and K). They are found in butter, margarine, meat, vegetable oils, etc.

5. *Minerals* help build blood, bones, and teeth and aid in vital body functions. Calcium is a mineral that is often neglected by adults. Even though your bones are no longer growing, your body needs calcium because it can be withdrawn from the bones if your food does not provide enough to meet your needs. Calcium is also needed for normal blood clotting and for healthy nerve and muscle action. Unless you drink two 8-ounce glasses of milk or eat 3 ounces of cheese every day, you are not getting enough calcium. You don't need to worry about milk causing excessive mucus production—there is no scientific evidence to show that it does!

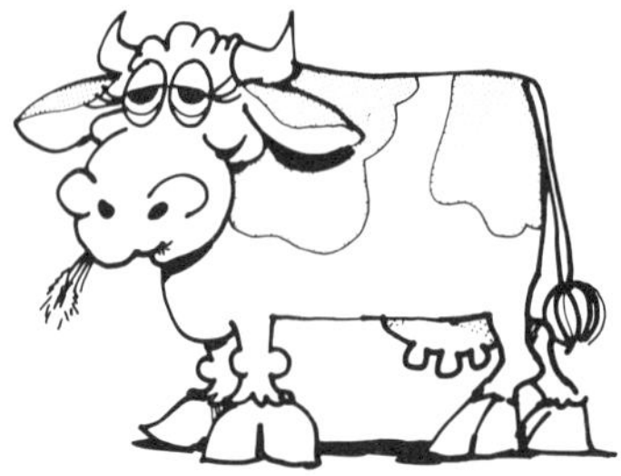

Iron is a mineral that is required for healthy blood and is often neglected in our diets. Liver is the best source of iron but it is also available in eggs, other meats, fish, whole grains, poultry, and dried fruits such as raisins.

6. *Vitamins* are essential for proper utilization of food and for healthy functioning of the body. Practically everything that goes on within our bodies requires the action of one or more vitamins.

Vitamin A is necessary for normal growth, good vision, and to fight infection. It is found in butter and dark, leafy green and yellow vegetables.

The B vitamins are necessary for nerve function, digestion, good appetite, and healthy skin. Whole-grain breads and cereals, meat, poultry, fish, nuts, and dairy products are the best sources of the B vitamins.

The amount of vitamin C needed is controversial. The best sources of vitamin C are the citrus fruits (oranges and grapefruit), papaya, strawberries, broccoli, and turnip greens. Be sure to eat two or three servings of these foods every day.

Vitamin E is another vitamin surrounded by controversy as to the amount needed and what it can do for us. If you are considering supplementing your diet, check with your doctor first. The best food source of vitamin E is wheat germ. Other good sources are vegetable oils, nuts, and legumes.

When making your food selections, keep in mind that you will get more nutrition for your money from foods that come directly from nature. In other words, 5 pounds of oranges cost about as much as a box of cookies; a 10-pound bag of potatoes costs less than a box of instant dehydrated mashed potatoes; and a quart of milk costs much less than a six-pack of a cola drink.

Eating right is important for anyone, but it is extremely important for COPD patients. Not only should you eat a well-balanced diet, but you must also follow special nutritional guidelines because of your disease. Some nutritional problems and ways to overcome them are listed in the following section.

Distension

Eating too much at one time or eating certain foods can cause your stomach to become "bloated" (distended), limiting motion of your diaphragm and making it harder for you to breathe.

SOLUTION

1. Eat six small meals a day instead of three big ones. This is a good idea for another reason. Digesting food takes energy, which requires oxygen, so eating small meals uses up less oxygen.
2. Avoid the gas-forming foods which cause you discomfort. Some people are bothered by:

Brussels sprouts	Apples
Cabbage	Watermelon
Broccoli	Cantaloupe
Sauerkraut	Honeydew melon
Cauliflower	Some fruit juices
Asparagus	Onions
Beans	Radishes
Carbonated beverages	Beer
Excessive sweets	

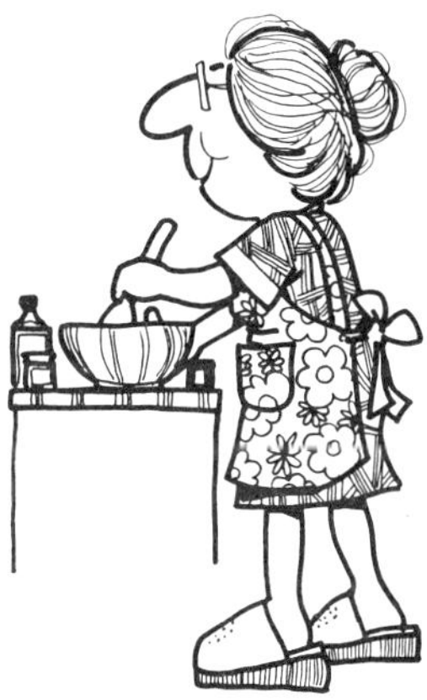

3. Eat slowly, in a leisurely, relaxed atmosphere. If you rush through the meal or talk and chew at the same time, you might swallow air. Take time to enjoy your meals.
4. If the feeling of fullness continues from one meal to the next, you will need to eat food that leaves the stomach as quickly as possible. Fatty

foods and fried foods should be avoided since they take longer to leave the stomach.

5. You can further reduce the volume of food in the stomach by taking liquids 1 hour *before* and 1 hour *after,* rather than *during,* the meal.

Loss of muscle mass

Because of the decreased activity of many patients with lung disease, their muscles become weak and flabby. Then when they feel good enough to do something, they are too weak.

SOLUTION

1. Eat a well-balanced diet to get the proper vitamins and minerals.
2. Eat more high-protein foods such as meat, fish, poultry, dairy products.
3. You can boost the protein and calorie content of your diet without greatly increasing the amount of food consumed. High-protein food additives, such as nonfat dry milk, may be added to sauces, gravies, creamed dishes, casseroles, puddings, custards, meatloaf, etc.; you can add up to 1/4 cup of the dry milk to many recipes without altering the flavor.
4. Make "double-strength" milk by adding nonfat dry milk to regular whole milk, then mix well and chill.
5. Use milk, preferably "double-strength," instead of water for cooking cereals, diluting canned cream soups, mixing puddings, and making instant cocoa.
6. Add small pieces of cooked meat to canned soups and to casseroles.
7. Add grated cheese to vegetables, casseroles, and cream sauces.
8. Spread cream cheese or peanut butter on toast, whole wheat bread, apple slices, fresh pears, or celery.
9. Use yogurt for a dressing for fruit salads. Cottage cheese and cream cheese make good combinations with fruit salads.
10. Add hard-cooked eggs to tuna and chicken, for either sandwiches or salads. Finely chopped egg may be added to sauces and some casseroles without altering the flavor.

Loss of appetite

Increased mucus production and some of the medications you take can result in appetite loss.

SOLUTION

1. Take medicines with milk or meals.
2. Do bronchial drainage, IPPB, or exercising at least 1 hour before or after meals.

3. Drink a small glass of wine (not too much) before eating one meal.
4. Prepare foods with enticing aromas and vary your menus.
5. Food that is attractively served in a pleasant atmosphere is more tempting.
   a. Vary the colors and textures of food that is served.
   b. Use garnishes to brighten your plate.
   c. Colorful table settings, soft background music, and/or a change of location (a patio or sunny park) may make mealtime more enjoyable.
6. Get some fresh air and light exercise a short time before your meal.
7. Share a meal with a friend. Happy thoughts and pleasant feelings will help you enjoy your meal more and improve your appetite.

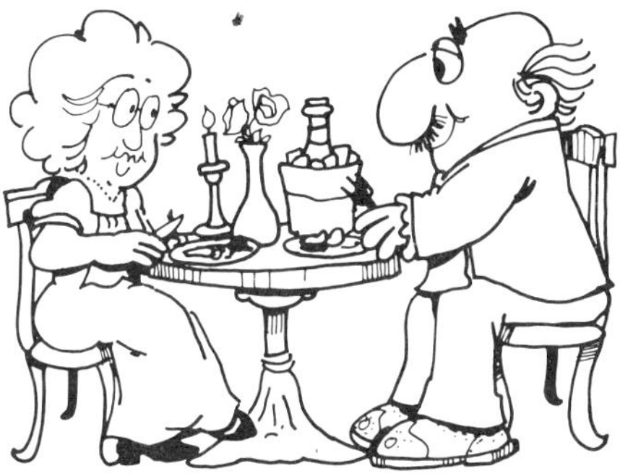

8. Take advantage of meals available at community centers, churches, and neighborhood schools. Call the American Lung Association, local health department, YMCA, or local church for locations near you.

Hydration

Keeping secretions thin and easy to bring up is *very important*. If you do not drink enough fluids, your secretions will be thick and sticky and become a good breeding place for infections.

SOLUTION

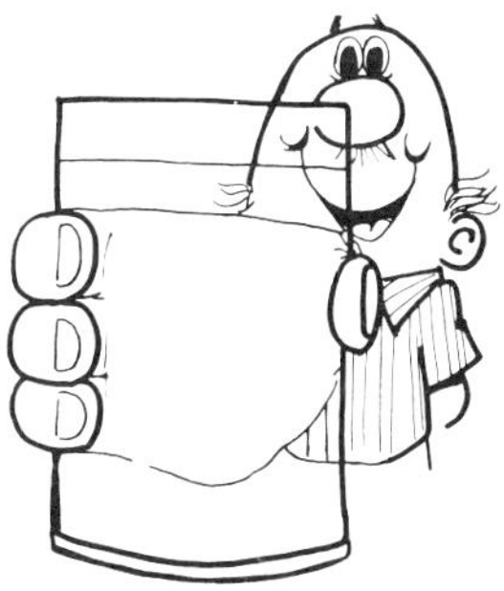

1. Drink at least 1½ quarts of liquid each day. Besides water, you can drink fruit juices, nectars, milkshakes, and so on.
2. Check for dehydration (too little fluid) by watching for color changes in your urine. If your urine becomes a deeper yellow, you will need to increase your intake of fluids. Urine color varies among individuals, de-

pending on medication, vitamins, and so on; but it is nearly colorless when the fluid intake is high.

3. When you are infected, have a fever, or the weather is very hot, increase your fluid intake to 2 or $2^1/_2$ quarts per day.

Potassium depletion

If you take water pills (diuretics), you not only lose fluid but also potassium. When your potassium level is low, you might notice such symptoms as weakness, tingling, numbness of the fingers, or leg cramps. Low potassium level is also present in some COPD patients who are not taking medication.

SOLUTION

Eat several high-potassium foods every day.

High-potassium foods

Bananas	Peanuts	Beef
Oranges	Yams	Dry skim milk
Orange juice	Avocados	Winter squash
Raisins	Broccoli	Brussels sprouts
Dried apricots	Tomatoes	Pork
Dates	Potatoes	Chicken
Prunes	Fresh spinach	Fish
Cooked dried beans	Fresh mushrooms	Milk

Low-salt diet

Sometimes eating salt, even normal amounts, may cause you to retain excess fluid in your body. Your doctor will tell you if your condition, or certain medicines you take, may lead to this problem with salt. If the problem is not too great, just avoiding the salt shaker in cooking and at the table is often enough salt restriction. If your problem is more severe, you may need to avoid all salty foods (ham, luncheon meats, bacon, canned soups, snack foods, and convenience foods). Your doctor will tell you how much your salt intake should be restricted and your dietitian will provide a specific low-salt diet to meet your needs.

TIPS TO SAVE TIME AND ENERGY

Meal preparation can be a real drain on your energy and leave you without the strength you need to enjoy your meal. The following solutions may be helpful:

1. One-dish meals (casseroles) are easy to prepare and clean up.
2. Prepare recipes in larger quantities and freeze individual portions for reheating.

3. Make up your own "TV dinners" with leftover single servings, but don't rely on commercial TV dinners. Their nutritive value is less than what you prepare yourself and they are very high in sodium.
4. Avoid the last-minute rush. Meal preparation is less tiring when some of the meal is partly or fully prepared in advance, such as the salad, dessert, or a casserole.
5. Oven cooking is less tiring than stove-top cooking. You might also try a slow cooker or crock pot.

SUPPLEMENTAL VITAMINS

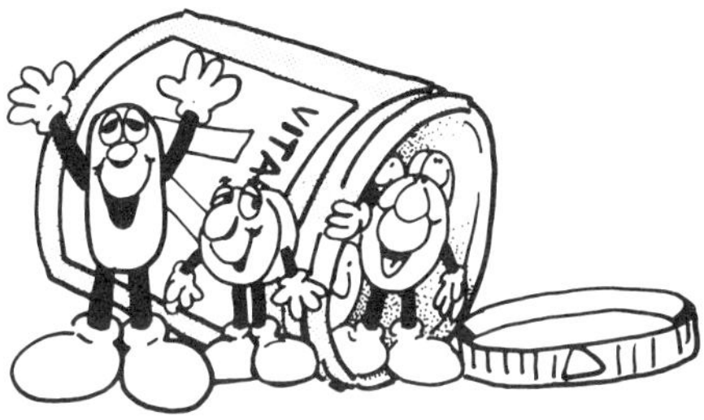

Large doses of vitamins and minerals are not recommended, but when food intake is limited it might be necessary to take a daily vitamin/mineral supplement. It is particularly difficult to get the recommended amount of iron from the food you eat, so be sure your supplement includes it. Check with your doctor for his recommendations.

Good luck! **Good health!** **Good eating!**

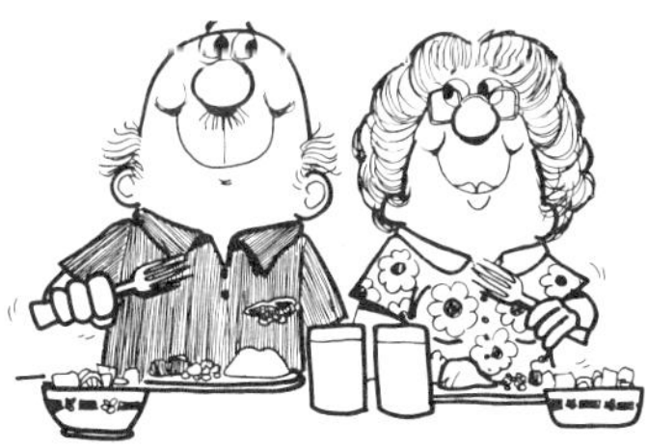

12 You don't have to be grounded

Travel is an important part of life for most people. You may need to travel for business purposes, to visit with family and friends, or just to enjoy "getting away" and seeing new places (or happy old ones). But when you have a breathing problem, the thought of leaving the security of home may prevent you from venturing out. Questions of safety, getting sick, and needing help arise. For most patients with COPD, however, there are relatively few contraindications to travel. With a little foresight and determination, you don't have to be grounded!

The most crucial consideration is that while *you* can take a vacation, there is *no* vacation from respiratory care. You cannot tell your lungs that you are going on a trip and will return in 2 weeks. Although your daily routine will be interrupted, you must adhere as closely as possible to your respiratory care routine. This means you must take your medications regularly and maintain hydration; if your routine includes bronchial drainage and breathing and physical training exercises, they must be continued.

The most important move you can make in planning a happy and healthy vacation is to consult your doctor. He will review your therapy and indicate whether any part of your program can be modified while you are away. He may want to give you the name of a physician at your destination whom you can contact if any difficulties arise. He may even want to send a copy of your medical records ahead.

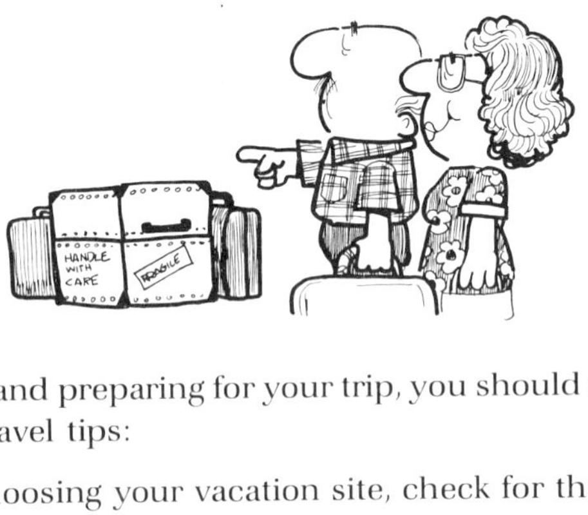

In planning and preparing for your trip, you should consider some of the following travel tips:

TIP 1. When choosing your vacation site, check for the following:
Infections. Are there any viral flu epidemics at your destination?

(Of course, you should check with your doctor about obtaining a yearly flu vaccine, regardless of known epidemics.) Does anyone you are going to visit have a cold? If so, you may want to postpone your trip.

Air pollution. How smoggy is the area? Will you have an air-conditioned room?

Allergy. If allergies play a part in your illness, avoid areas that have high pollen counts.

Altitude. Consider the altitude of the area. As we ascend, air becomes less dense and there is less oxygen available to us. At short distances above sea level this change is insignificant. But in cities at very high altitudes (that is, over 1 mile [5280 feet] high), or during air flight (the cabins are pressurized to an atmosphere equal to 1 mile high), the effect upon people with COPD may be important, resulting in increased shortness of breath and other symptoms.

TIP **2.** Make a checklist of your medications. Take enough to last you through the trip and for a few extra days in case of delay. It is occasionally difficult to get prescriptions filled from one state to another; nevertheless, obtain extra prescriptions from your physician as another safeguard.

TIP **3.** When traveling to foreign countries, you may need a supply of general medicine (aspirin, antidiarrhea medicine, and others) with you. The quality of medications is not the same throughout the world. Avoid unknown medications, especially "over-the-counter" preparations, as many of these contain substances that can cause harm. Be very sure to take a sufficient supply of your prescription medications if you are going to a foreign country.

TIP **4.** Establish a travel routine for your treatments, exercise, and cleaning of equipment. Write it down and follow it carefully.

TIP **5.** Travel is tiring: allow time for frequent rest stops. Relax and enjoy yourself. Don't try to do too much in one day; get adequate sleep.

TIP **6.** Discuss with your doctor how different altitude changes may affect you. If you need supplemental oxygen at higher altitudes, you must take it with you or arrange to have it there when you arrive.

TIP **7.** If your doctor says that you will need supplemental oxygen while flying, contact the airline in advance. Most airlines *won't* let you bring your own equipment on board. They *will* supply oxygen for you for the duration of the trip. Some airlines won't allow oxygen use at all. Others require a written release, from your doctor, to travel and information on the amount of oxygen to be used. A few even require accompaniment by a medical person or friend. So check the rules well in advance.

TIP **8.** If you use oxygen or other respiratory equipment, ask your local vendor for the name of a company that could assist you at your destination. You may have to take some of your equipment with you, but you can arrange for whatever equipment and oxygen supplies you need to be waiting for you upon your arrival. (Don't forget your cleaning supplies!)

TIP **9.** Go prepared for climate and weather changes—extra clothes for warmth, and so on.

TIP **10.** Avoid smoking areas whenever possible, whether traveling by plane or train.

• • •

Travel makes life interesting and rewarding. Travel whenever possible, but plan ahead.

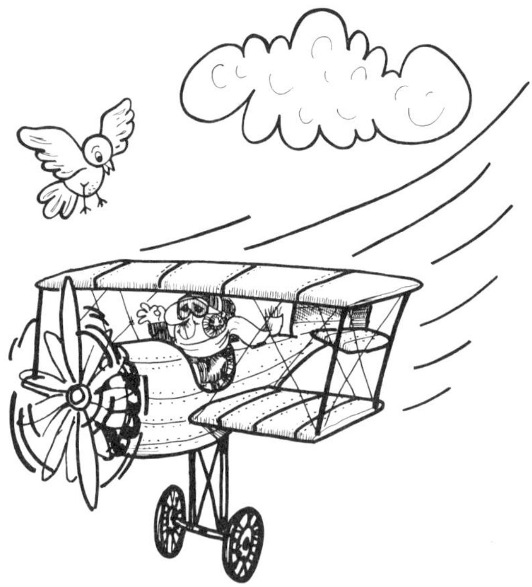

13 Smoking, smog, and other bad stuff

SMOKING

Today just about everybody—even those who continue their smoking habit—knows that cigarettes may produce severe and lingering health effects. The most serious effects involve the heart and lungs. People who smoke have an increased risk of developing coronary heart disease and having a heart attack. The potential effects on the lungs are multiple.

For example, smoking can paralyze the hair-like cilia in the bronchial walls. As a result, these cilia cannot do their job of moving contaminated mucus toward the throat, where it can be eliminated easily. Mucus collects in the bronchial tubes and clogs up the bronchi, impairing movement of air and making the lungs more susceptible to infection.

Smoking also irritates the mucous cells of the bronchi, stimulating them to produce excess mucus. This may further clog the lungs and lead to chronic cough, in an effort to clear the bronchi of mucus. In addition, smoking may cause the lining of the bronchial tubes to swell and become narrowed. This narrowing makes breathing more difficult and cough less effective.

Cigarette smoking is not the only risk factor in chronic lung disease. Other factors, such as a deficiency of an enzyme in the blood, alpha-1-antitrypsin, can predispose a person to the development of emphysema. Smoking, however, is by far the most important risk factor.

Lung cancer is another problem linked to smoking. Cancer-causing elements, known as *carcinogens,* are found in cigarette smoke. These chemical agents may cause normal cells to develop into cancerous ones. Statistically, smokers have a far greater chance of developing cancer of the lungs than nonsmokers. Lung cancer has been a leading cause of death among American males for some years. Recently, the number of women with this disease has increased as they take up the smoking habit.

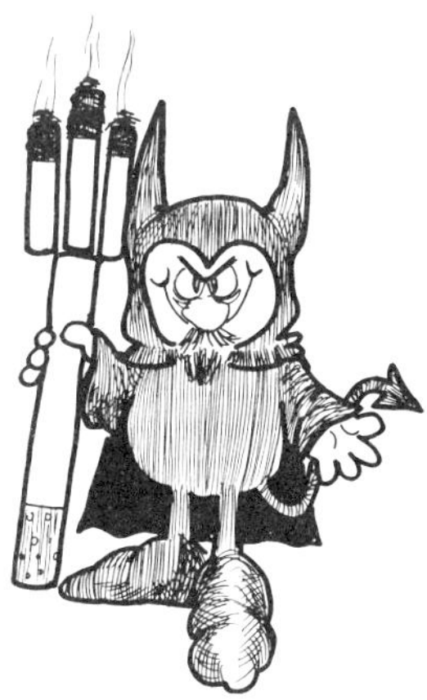

People with lung disease who persist in their smoking—of cigarettes or any other tobacco product—are engaging in behavior that must be curtailed if treatments administered by the doctor are to be of maximum benefit. Every cigarette that you smoke may harm your lungs more. If you smoke, make every effort to *quit!*

The benefits derived from giving up the smoking habit are great. You may actually improve your lung condition! The risk of heart disease, cancer, and the development of further lung disease may be reduced. Coughing episodes and mucus production will decrease. Your ability to breathe will improve, thereby reducing the disability from your lung disease. It's worth it!!

ENVIRONMENTAL EXPOSURE

Your breathing may be affected by a variety of factors found in the environment, for example, temperature and humidity. These factors may affect some people but not others; that is, the response to a certain environment is highly individual. Since we are all affected differently, it would follow that there is no such thing as an "ideal" climate or environment for all COPD patients. The environment in which you feel most comfortable is the best for you. Let's look at some of the environmental factors that may influence your breathing.

Second-hand smoke

Unfortunately, you may be bothered by smoking even though you've given up the habit. This can happen when you are exposed to the smoke generated by others. Although the degree of irritation is much less than that caused by personal smoking, inhalation of "second-hand" smoke may result in more shortness of breath. If this is the case, you should steer clear of contaminated air. Also, don't be afraid to tell others that their smoking is bothering you. Telling friends, "Yes, I mind if you smoke!" is especially difficult at first. But with a little practice, you can manage. Here are some pointers. Be polite. Many smokers are not aware of the discomfort you may experience and will respect your request. Placing a "No Smoking" sign on your door or desk may be all that is necessary with friends. If you occasionally meet with a hostile response, remember that these people are probably not any nicer about this than they are about anything else. Seek out well-ventilated restaurants, or "No Smoking" areas in restaurants and other public places. But avoid panic when exposed to smoke; that can be worse than any effect of smoke itself. Work yourself, and with others, to educate smokers about how you feel and why your desire for a "non-smoke" environment should be honored.

Air pollution

Research suggests that some people with asthma, chronic bronchitis, and emphysema may have more trouble breathing, and increased coughing, on days of heavy air pollution. If you are bothered by air pollution, you may want to check the pollution levels before venturing out. The four major pollutants are sulfates, ozone, particulates, and carbon monoxide, primarily from factories and automobile exhaust. Carbon monoxide, from car exhaust, interferes with the blood's ability to carry oxygen. When this dirty air is exposed to the hot sun, it gets even more irritating.

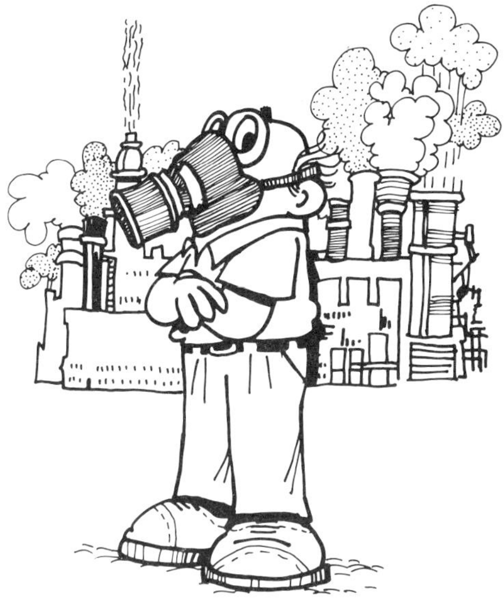

If you are bothered by pollution, avoid it when you travel. Avoid heavy exertion on days when pollution is severe. Air conditioning in your house (or motel or hotel when away) may help. Avoid rush-hour traffic, when automobile exhaust pollution is worst.

Industrial pollution

This occurs when the air in your place of work bothers your breathing. Your breathing may be affected by dusts, fumes, and gases and vapors from chemicals. There are some well-known kinds of industrial pollution like exposure to asbestos or coal dust; but often the exposure is unreported. We are discovering new forms every day. Therefore, if the air in your work place bothers you, you need to do something about it. See what dust and fumes might be produced in your work place. If possible, have them eliminated—at least, have ventilation improved. It may take some "detective work," but it needs to be done.

Temperature

Some people are affected by temperature. Very cold air has been known to cause bronchospasm. Temperatures over 90° F can also affect your breathing and cause dehydration.

Wet vs. dry climates

The only person who can tell if a wet or dry climate is better for your breathing is *you*. You should visit both climates and decide.

Allergy

True allergies are abnormal responses to materials that exist in the environment. For example, onions make everyone's eyes water; that is not an allergy but an *irritation*. It is sometimes difficult to distinguish between irritation and true allergy. If you sneeze, develop a runny nose, have itching eyes or wheezing on exposure to things *that cause no symptoms in others* (for example, flowers, cats, or certain foods), you may have an allergy. Obviously, the best thing to do about allergies is to avoid them when possible. When avoidance isn't possible, allergies can be controlled with medicines such as antihistamines and corticosteroids. Most people with COPD (usually asthmatics) know their allergies and live with them.

It would be nice if we could escape to an environment that is "ideal" for everyone. But since we can't, we must each learn to make the one we have as healthy as possible.

14 The psychology of better breathing

If a man does not keep pace with his companions,
perhaps it is because he hears a different drummer.

H. D. Thoreau

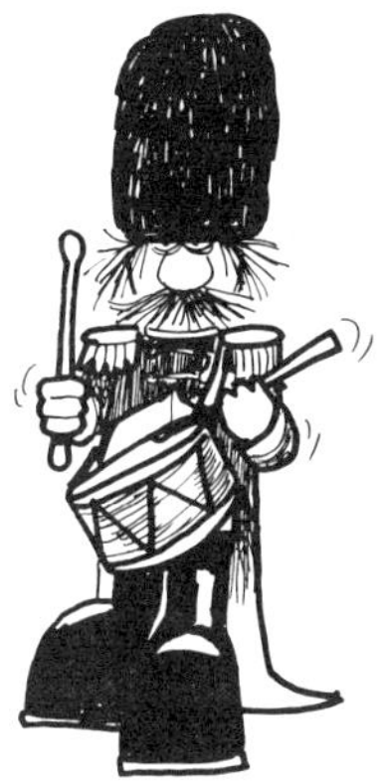

All of us would like to be able to do *what* we want, *when* we want to do it, and *how* we want to do it. Unfortunately, we learn that many factors impose limitations. How we deal with these limitations determines how happy, productive, and pleasant our lives are.

Our state of health is one factor that can impose a significant limitation; and any chronic illness, such as COPD, imposes those limits permanently. A chronic limit can be particularly difficult to deal with and can make individuals angry, anxious, and depressed. While this is understandable, it is unfortunate because the mind and body are closely interrelated. That is, physical health can influence mental health—and vice versa. This is particularly true for patients with COPD. Emotions can influence breathing in people with *normal* lungs; they can have *major* effects on breathing when COPD is present. Therefore, dealing with your emotional or psychological self is very important to your physical health.

Saying "Deal with your emotions" or "Learn how to live with limitations" is easy; *doing* it is difficult. This chapter may help you to do so by explaining the emotional problems common to patients with COPD.

In the main, there are two kinds of problems you may face: how you view *yourself* and how you relate to *others.*

YOU—THE PERSON WITH COPD

We all have a certain "image" of ourselves physically and emotionally. That image is critical to how we function and to how we relate to others because our self-esteem is based upon it. COPD may be associated with a number of changes in physical image. You may gain weight because of inactivity or steroid medications; or you may lose weight because of decreased appetite. You may have noisy breathing, or you may cough and produce sputum. You may have to walk and do other things more slowly. You may need to use oxygen "in public." All of these things may impair your physical image and cause you to feel unattractive and odd. If *you* feel this way, you may think that others see you the same way, and your self-esteem will suffer. The first thing to recognize is that other people have a lot to think about besides how you look and breathe. If they do notice and ask questions, such curiosity on their part is normal. It can be satisfied by telling them the truth. You can calmly say, "It's all right, I have a lung condition and need to use oxygen"; or "It makes me cough more than I would like." Most people understand and will easily accept the truth—and you. The people who "count" will accept individuals for what they are, not how they look. People who wear casts on their legs are *always* asked "What happened?" A straight answer ends the curiosity and normal interpersonal relationships resume.

Another limitation that can bother people with COPD is their vulnerability to things over which they have no direct control. All of us are vulnerable to a number of outside forces. But with COPD, many factors may pose a special threat to well-being: for example, infectious agents, atmospheric conditions, and environmental pollutants. Such factors may lead to unpredictable changes in daily activities, which is irritating if you are used to being organized and to carefully planning your daily activities.

COPD may lead to other alterations which can impair self-esteem. You may need to modify your work schedule or seek early retirement. You may need to modify or eliminate certain pleasurable activities: tennis, golfing, bowling, climbing, and other forms of recreation. You may explore a change in geography to seek a more favorable climate, causing you to leave behind friends and familiar surroundings. These changes can cause periods of depression, which practically all patients with COPD experience.

Depression involves feelings of sadness, hopelessness, and worthlessness. The symptoms are subtle in the beginning, consisting of a lack of interest in things (including your personal appearance, food, outside activities) and fatigue. "Going out" becomes a chore, friends and hobbies are dropped. Everything becomes "too much effort." Depression needs to be recognized early. Unless it is, inactivity results that can worsen your condition. There is no easy antidote. You must force yourself to start moving, call friends, and go out; and, if necessary, seek outside counseling.

Certain phobias (abnormal fears of common experiences) may develop because of the real fear of becoming short of breath. For example, panic may be associated with entering closed spaces, even a shower stall. This panic worsens shortness of breath and a terrifying vicious cycle of fear and further difficulty in breathing can result. This cycle can be prevented by learning how to control such situations with proper relaxation and breathing techniques.

Another common response to COPD (or any chronic illness) is denial. It is certainly useful to avoid becoming totally preoccupied with yourself and your illness. But denying illness can be hazardous, if it leads to forgetting medicines, treatments, doctor's appointments, and real limits on your activity. It may lead to hiding your limitations from other people. You need to strike a balance between living with your limitations and denying their existence.

HOW YOU RELATE TO OTHERS: THE SPOUSE

Pulmonary illness has an impact not only upon you, but upon the others in your immediate family because it often alters the roles you play in relationship to others. For example, in marriage each partner usually accepts certain responsibilities. Each partner comes to rely on the other for certain activities: one may deal with finances and with social arrangements; one may deal more effectively with certain problems or people or with house maintenance or shopping. When pulmonary illness occurs, the nature of this sharing may need to change, temporarily or permanently. The spouse may have to assume *new* roles. There is danger in this situation for both patient and spouse. The patient may become more and more dependent on the healthier spouse (who, in turn, may become essentially a full-time nurse). The one with COPD may fear being left alone and require more and more from the spouse, including giving up his or her outside activities and work. Both resent (often quietly) the situation—one angry about being dependent, the other angry about becoming so depended-upon. The answer is to discuss what is going on in the marriage. Excessive dependence (or doting) is to be discouraged. Both partners should do their share, even if those shares are modified in amount or nature.

SEX

In order to maintain an active, enjoyable sexual life there are also certain changes that a couple may have to make when one member has pulmonary illness. They may not be able to perform some of their previous sexual practices since the extent of exercise tolerance may be diminished. The length of time spent in activities such as foreplay may have to be modified. In addition, certain positions used during intercourse may no longer be comfortable and a change may be necessary. But there is no way that modifications can be made in sexual activity unless the couple is open enough to *talk about* sex. An unfortunate type of communication that couples frequently engage in is a game called "I hope you can read my mind." That is, one partner wishes something changed sexually and hopes that the spouse will comply with the *unspoken* wish. The ice may have to be broken by one person just coming out and talking about it. As an example, one patient was required to use oxygen for any type of exertion, including sexual activity. She felt that having her oxygen tank in the bedroom detracted from the sexual atmosphere during relations with her husband. Her solution was to place the tank outside the bedroom and use a long tube that reached the bed. There is no reason for sexual activity to stop because a person has pulmonary illness. The key is to be open about it, and modify the activity to that which is physically possible.

FRIENDS

If you have a negative image of yourself, it may interfere with your friendships. You may begin to fear that you are "more trouble than you are worth," that you are a burden to others. Your response may be to withdraw from relationships or to try and maintain a facade (doing more than you should really do). Again, the fact is that your friends rarely share your feelings (that you are a "burden") and will respect and understand your limits. If you ask them to walk slower, or not smoke around you, or alter social plans, almost all will understand and respond. But you can't play "read my mind." You must tell them of your limits, not hide them. You can take an active role in planning your social life so that it fits within your limitations. There is no need to be totally left out.

THE "BOTTOM LINE"

We have reviewed some of the common problems faced by patients with pulmonary illness and some of the feelings they may develop. There are some very important principles to remember to help you maintain both a positive state of mental health and a positive quality of life. First, having a pulmonary illness does not necessarily mean you must "give up" certain activities in your life. Instead you should *modify* the activity and still be involved in it. Many people have difficulty learning to "pace" themselves; but with patience and practice, it can be done. For example, patients who are distraught that they can no longer play 18 holes of golf find that it is possible to play 9 holes with a cart. Patient and spouse can enjoy golf again, a pleasure they thought was gone forever. When you have pulmonary illness, you may develop misconceptions as to the safe limits of physical exertion; that is, once you begin to develop shortness of breath, you may *stop* the activity instead of slowing it down. There is a tendency to stop sooner and sooner in the activity, and consequently, to begin to feel that you can do very little. Although you may have to slow down, you can learn that if you "push" yourself a little, you can do more than you thought. Doing more will improve your self-

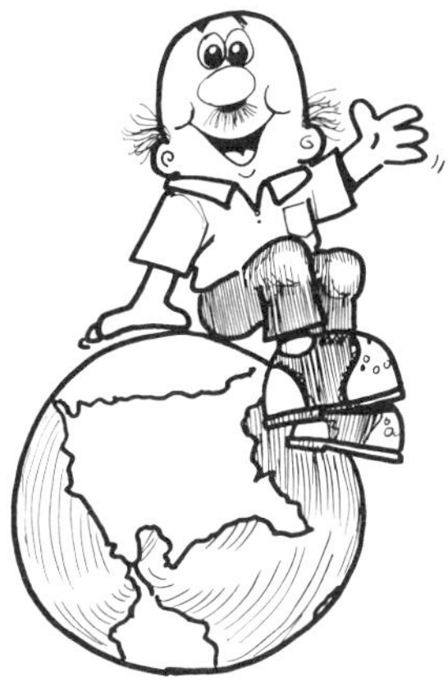

esteem and endurance. The important thing is to figure out *how* you can do what you like. Don't give it up! Rearrange it! Adapt it to you! Soon the pace will no longer be planned; it will become natural to you. You can continue to be involved with the world, with your family, and with your friends.

Another important principle is to learn as much as possible about your illness. You should try to learn about your lung function, your medicines, and your treatments. Ask questions of doctors, nurses, therapists, and other patients until answers have been obtained. The process of education concerning your illness has an enormous psychological value. As you know more about your illness, some of the unfounded fears can be dispelled. In addition, as you develop more understanding, you can play a more active role in keeping yourself healthy and helping yourself when you are ill. A great deal can be learned not only from medical personnel, but from other patients as well. People with COPD have accumulated a vast amount of experience about how to live successfully within the physical limits that exist. You can share their experiences, contribute your own, and give each other support. This can be done through rehabilitation programs, American Lung Association meetings, and in informal groups.

The essence of good psychological health is to maintain a positive attitude toward living, while knowing the facts and being realistic. Remain as active as possible, and try to maintain your sense of humor. Your life is not "over" with pulmonary illness—it is *changed,* but you can enjoy this changed life greatly if you maintain a positive image of yourself.

15 When to call your doctor and what to do in an emergency

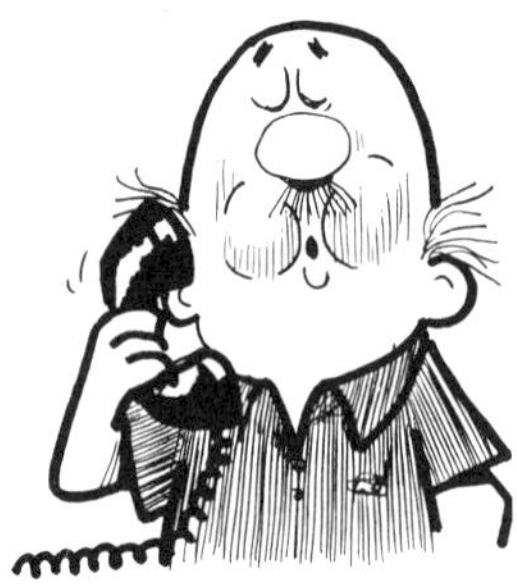

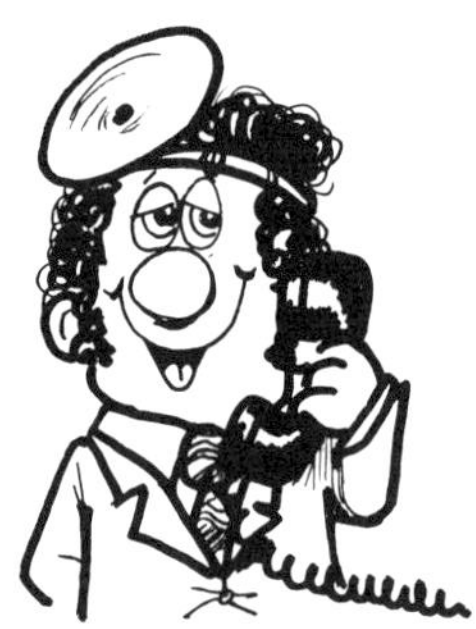

Most COPD patients have regularly scheduled visits with their doctor. But when should you call him between these visits? Usually, in discussions with your doctor, signals are worked out to cover this question. In general, however, there are two major "signals" that your doctor will want to know about: (1) any *change* in your symptoms, particularly if this change lasts more than 1 day; (2) any *new* symptoms that you develop. Obviously, we all have our ups and downs, our good days and bad. But changes and new symptoms should be called to your doctor's attention.

Some of the *changes* or *new symptoms* that might be important are:

- Fever
- Increased shortness of breath, difficulty in breathing, wheezing (more than usual)
- Increased coughing (more frequent, more severe, or both)
- Increased sputum production
- Change in color of sputum (to yellow, gray, or green)
- Change in consistency of sputum (thicker)
- Swelling in ankles, legs, or around eyes
- Sudden weight gain (3 to 5 pounds overnight)
- Palpitations of the heart or faster pulse than usual
- Unusual dizziness, sleepiness, headaches, visual disturbances, irritability, trouble thinking
- Loss of appetite (more than usual)
- Dehydration evidenced by concentrated urine and dryness of skin
- Chest pains
- Blood in sputum, urine, or bowel movement

You should discuss these "signals" with your doctor. He may want you to change your medicines or add new one(s) if they develop (for example, to increase fluid intake and/or to start a preselected antibiotic for fever and increased cough). The more you work out these signals ahead of time, the better you will be able to deal with these changes, and the less frequently you will have to call your doctor on an emergency basis. **But when in doubt, check it out with your doctor.**

WHAT TO DO IN AN EMERGENCY

Many patients and their spouses and/or family members want to know what to do in an emergency. There are two things that will make it rather simple to deal with this question: (1) become familiar with the options for medical care open to you, and have a plan; (2) become familiar with what an "emergency" is.

In general, an "emergency" is some *sudden* change or *new* development in your condition, particularly changes or new things that impair your ability to function or that frighten you. Sudden and/or severe chest pains or shortness of breath are the most common "emergencies" in COPD patients. Coughing up blood is another. So *sudden* changes in your condition and *new symptoms* of a major kind usually constitute a true emergency.

Of course, many patients with lung disease have mild changes that are frightening and may cause panic. Other sections of this book offer methods for dealing with panic. For example, if breathing becomes more difficult, you should assume a sitting position and lean forward slightly; pursed lip breathing usually helps, as may using relaxation techniques (see Chapter 9). Inhalation of a bronchodilator aerosol (see Chapter 4) is useful if the shortness of breath is caused by bronchospasm. You must learn how to deal with such episodes; discussions with your doctor about these and other maneuvers will help.

But what if the symptoms are severe, don't go away, or are new? This constitutes a true emergency. In this situation, most patients want to see their doctor *immediately*, and that is a good idea because he knows you best. But that may not be possible or even in your best interests in an emergency. The key to making an emergency plan is, again, a discussion with your doctor. You should determine: when he is available (no one is available 24 hours a day, 7 days a week!); how you can contact him; and, if he is not available when you try to contact him, what you should do. Many doctors have associates who "take calls" when they themselves are not available; some do not. If you cannot contact him (or his associates), what should you do: call an ambulance or the "paramedics"? If you do that, to what emergency facility should you be taken?

The answers to these questions will be different in different communities. In general, an "emergency" means you need prompt access to medical care. Obviously, it is an advantage if your doctor (or his associates) is available to provide your medical history, even if he cannot be physically present.

Therefore, the important thing is to *plan* ahead so you know what to do. Have a written "plan" near the telephone—names of *whom* to call and the proper telephone numbers: your primary doctor, "backup" doctor(s), ambulance or paramedic numbers, location of the nearest emergency facility. Think through the situation ahead of time; put yourself in the place of your spouse or friend as if *you* were helping *them* in an emergency. Once you have a "plan," there is no reason for anyone to panic in an emergency. So "worry about it" now and get it worked out now. Hopefully, you will never need to put it into action!

Many patients don't want to "bother" their doctor; but whether your symptoms warrant "bothering" your doctor should be decided by the doctor. As you get to know each other and you become more knowledgeable, this decision will become easier. But err on the side of "bothering" whenever you are uncertain.

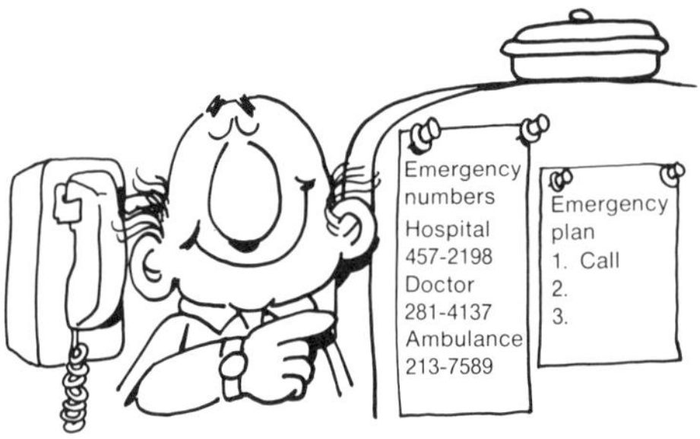

16 Getting it all together

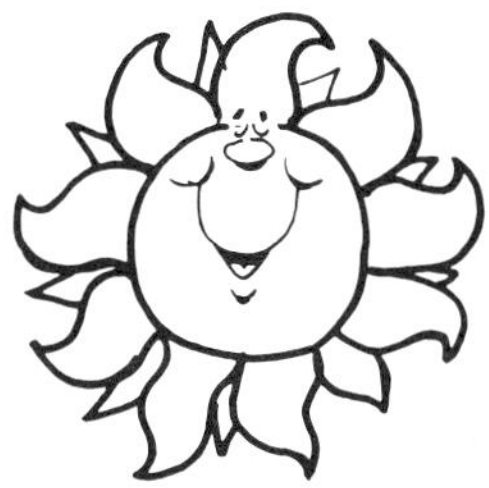

Now that you have been introduced to the various methods of handling your COPD, you must learn to fit them into 1 day. Writing out a daily schedule is one method of helping you develop a *workable,* balanced regimen of treatments, rest, exercise, and recreation. Start by listing what you need to do each day. All the key elements of *your* particular program should be included whether they consist of medications alone or include such things as bronchial drainage, breathing exercises, aerosol treatments, body improvement exercises, walks, special meals, and so on.

The schedule should be set up realistically so that you can follow it with as little frustration as possible. You should remember that you will have to push yourself at times and you *will* have to work—but the rewards will be plentiful!

The sequence of your program is important. Here are some tips to remember in setting up your daily schedule:

Bronchial drainage (as you have learned in Chapter 8) should *never* be done on a full stomach. It should be done before meals or 1 hour after meals.

Medication (pills) to open your airways (bronchodilators) should be taken at least 1/2 hour *before* doing each bronchial drainage treatment. This will help to widen the airway and therefore drain the mucus more effectively.

Inhaled bronchodilators and *mist-producing machines* (nebulizer, IPPB, etc.) should be scheduled for use before the bronchial drainage treatment.

Never *exercise* or walk immediately after a meal. Wait for an hour or so; or do your exercises before the meal.

Remember to schedule *naps* and *rest* periods, as well as snacks and fluids, throughout the day!

An example of a "typical" daily schedule is shown on the following page. With the help of your doctor, nurse, or therapist, fill out the blank schedule form, using the example as a guide.

SAMPLE SCHEDULE

MORNING

1. After awakening, take bronchodilator medication (pill).
2. Use inhaled bronchodilator.
3. Do bronchial drainage immediately afterward.
4. Breakfast.
5. After an hour or so, walk at designated speed and time. (Practice breathing exercises while walking.)
6. Have a nutritious snack with glass of liquid.
7. Rest.
8. Liquids. (Space liquid intake throughout day and keep a careful record of amounts.)
9. After you feel rested, do body improvement exercise(s).

AFTERNOON

1. Lunch.
2. Medications.
3. After an hour or so, practice breathing exercises and relaxation technique in a quiet setting.
4. Walk at designated speed and time. (Remember breathing exercises while walking.)
5. Snack, with 1 glass of liquid.
6. Body improvement exercise(s).
7. Liquids.

EVENING

1. Dinner.
2. After an hour or so, walk again at designated speed and time.
3. Medications.
4. An hour or more before bedtime, use bronchodilator aerosol.
5. Do bronchial drainage immediately afterward.
6. Do body improvement exercise(s).

YOUR DAILY SCHEDULE

MORNING

1. ______________________________
2. ______________________________
3. ______________________________
4. ______________________________

5. ______________________________

6. ______________________________

AFTERNOON

1. ______________________________

2. ______________________________

3. ______________________________

4. ______________________________

5. ______________________________

6. ______________________________

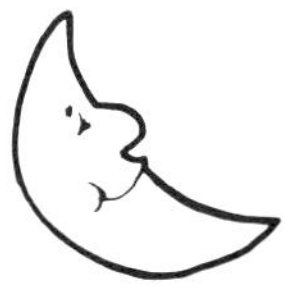

EVENING

1. ______________________________

2. ______________________________

3. ______________________________

4. ______________________________

5. ______________________________

6. ______________________________

17 A look to the future

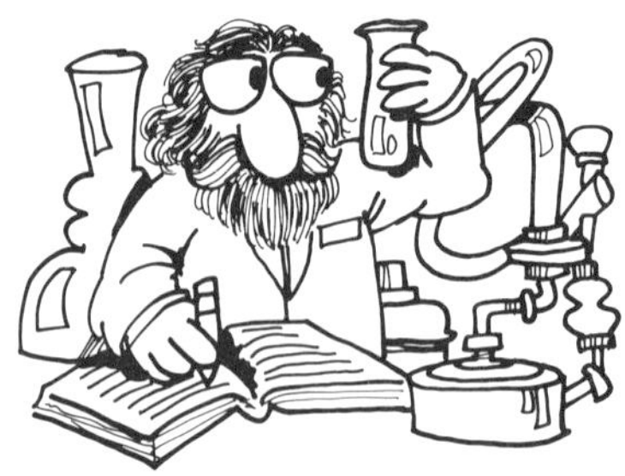

Medical research is constantly working toward the answers to many of the mysteries about COPD. With respect to emphysema, such research has indicated that the destruction of elastic tissue in the air sacs probably results from digestion of this tissue by an enzyme called *elastase.* This enzyme is normally carried around the body in the white blood cells. We also know that a blood protein called alpha-1-antitrypsin can inhibit (prevent, block) the effects of elastase. Some persons have an inherited deficiency of alpha-1-antitrypsin and get emphysema early in life, but this deficiency is rare. Why the elastase-inhibitor system becomes unbalanced in others is the object of intensive investigation.

The causes of chronic bronchitis also are being studied. Clearly, there is an association with cigarette smoking and certain industrial exposures—but why? What inhalants are responsible? What makes the bronchial tubes behave the way they do?

Existing drugs and treatments for all types of COPD are constantly being refined, and new ones developed. Just within the last few years, several new medicines have been introduced that relieve spasm of bronchial tubes or relieve inflammation of the mucous membrane. These are "better" than our older medicines in that they may either have fewer side effects or longer duration of action, are in a more convenient form to take, may prevent spasm (rather than treat it after it occurs), or may be more effective or less costly. While "new" does not mean "better" by any means (!), some of these "new" medicines may be "better" for you.

Another example of what lies ahead concerns drugs for better treatment of infection. Infections are caused by different kinds of invaders—bacteria, fungi, and viruses. Antibiotics are effective in treating infections caused by bacteria. Unfortunately, they are not very effective against fungi and not useful at all against viruses. No antibiotic can treat the flu and other virus infections. But research already has provided some drugs that can prevent (or treat) certain kinds of virus and fungus infections; and the future in this area looks bright.

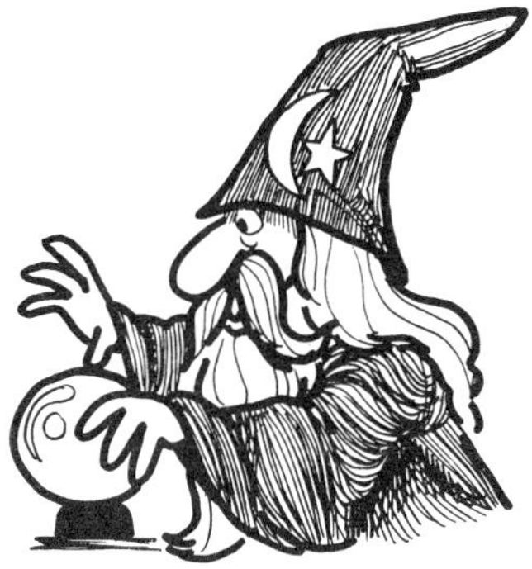

Some of the biggest gains are in education of the public about the factors that contribute to the disease. Young children are being taught the hazards of smoking in the hope that they will never begin to smoke. Smokers are being aided in their efforts to quit. Many agencies are working toward cleaning up our air, another source of lung pollution.

We are becoming aware of certain hazards to the lungs in the work place (with asbestos being the most famous), and are making progress in decreasing such hazards. Everywhere in our country, doctors and other medical personnel are becoming increasingly aware of COPD and are being trained in modern diagnosis and management.

The more that medical research discovers about COPD, the better doctors will be able to treat their patients. Since COPD is really several diseases, finding the key to each will be no easy task—but each breakthrough leads us closer to the answers. The ultimate goal is to learn enough so that COPD can be prevented.

Index